Homemade Keto Bread Cookbook

100 Low-Carb Ketogenic Bread Recipes to Kick your Carb Cravings

Tamara Milton

©Copyright 2020 by Cascade Publishing

All rights reserved.

It is not legal to reproduce, duplicate, or transmit any part of this document in either electronic means or in printed format. Recording of this publication is strictly prohibited.

Table Of Contents

INTRODUCTION	7
KETO DIET & KETO BREADS	8
So, What Actually Is The Ketogenic Diet?	10
Essential Keto Bread Ingredients	12
How To Make Perfect Keto Breads	14
CHAPTER 1 KETO BREAD LOAFS	15
Keto Blueberry Bread	17
Basic Keto Bread	18
Classic Coconut Bread	19
Classic Keto Bread	20
Mix Seed Almond Bread	21
Perky Pumpkin Bread	23
Keto Cornbread	24
Yogurt Cinnamon Bread	25
Keto Peanut Butter Bread	27
Super Cheese Bread	28
Almond Cream Bread	29
Peanut Cream Bread	30
Caraway Coconut Bread	31
Wonder Walnut Bread	33
Poppy Seed Bread	34
Keto Round Bread	35
Almond Olive Bread	36
Keto Flaxseed Bread	37
Coconut Mix Seed Bread	38
CHAPTER 2 SPECIAL KETO BREADS	39
All Time Favorite Garlic Bread	41

Keto Focaccia Bread	43
Keto Bacon Bread	44
Macadamia Magic Bread	45
Wholesome Broccoli Bread	46
Turmeric Baguette Bread	47
Almond Banana Bread	49
No-Flour Keto Egg Bread	50
Cauliflower Seeded Bread	51
Cheese & Bacon Bread	53
Zucchini Zeal Bread	54
Cashew Butter Bread	55
Jalapeno Delight Bread	56
Cream Onion Bread	57
Amazing Fougasse Bread	58
Keto Corn Bread	59
Walnut Zucchini Bread	61
Spinach Cheese Bread	63
Round Cream Bread	64
Cream Onion Keto Bread	65
Mug Mystery Bread	66

CHAPTER 3 KETO MUFFINS — 67

Chocolate Cream Muffins	68
Bacon Bake Muffins	69
Choco Pecan Muffins	70
Cinnamon Pumpkin Muffins	71
Almond Kale Muffins	73
Pumpkin Cinnamon Muffins	74
Keto Veggie Muffins	75
Sausage Oregano Muffins	76
Cranberry Spiced Muffins	77
Coconut Craving Muffins	79
Just Zucchini Muffins	80
Classic Keto Muffins	81
Hazelnut Muffins	82
Lemon Cream Muffins	83

Blueberry Keto Muffins … 85
Cinnamon Roll Muffins … 86

CHAPTER 4 KETO BUNS … 87

Almond Hamburger Buns … 88
Classic Sesame Buns … 89
Cheesy Hamburger Buns … 90
Garlic Keto Buns … 91
Pumpkin Keto Buns … 92
Everyday Breakfast Buns … 93
Mix Seed Mystery Bagels … 94
Cheesy Bagels … 95

CHAPTER 5 KETO BREADS ROLLS … 97

Classic Dinner Rolls … 98
Zucchini Bread Rolls … 99
Round Bread Rolls … 100
Mozzarella Bread Rolls … 101
Classic Oregano Pizza Crust … 102
Mozzarella Pizza Crust … 104

CHAPTER 6 KETO BREADSTICKS … 105

Aromatic Cinnamon Breadsticks … 107
Italian Style Cheesy Breadsticks … 108
Coconut Cheese Breadsticks … 109
Cheesy Garlic Breadsticks … 110
Seeded Keto Breadsticks … 111
Cheese Burst Breadsticks … 112
Sesame Seed Breadsticks … 113
Broccoli Cheese Breadsticks … 115
Cheesy Cheddar Breadsticks … 116
Cauliflower Spice Breadsticks … 117

CHAPTER 7 KETO CAKES … 119

Cinnamon Bundt Cake … 120
Keto Milk Cake … 121

- Spiced Brownie Cake — 123
- Cacao Zucchini Cakes — 124
- Dessert Choco Cake — 125
- Keto Sweet Cheese — 126
- Pumpkin Almond Cake — 127
- Coconut Spiced Mug Cakes — 128
- Keto Spice Mug Cake — 129

CHAPTER 8 KETO CRACKERS — 131
- Goat Cheese Rosemary Crackers — 133
- Spinach Chili Crackers — 134
- Yummy Parmesan Crackers — 135
- Rosemary Almond Crackers — 137
- Savory Seed Crackers — 138

CHAPTER 9 KETO COOKIES — 139
- Cocolicious Cookies — 140
- Pumpkin Cookies — 141
- Chocolate Chip Cookies — 143
- Almond Cream Cookies — 144

CONCLUSION — 145

INTRODUCTION

Fighting off those carb cravings can be a real struggle and let's be honest, we all love a sneaky little treat every so often. We work so hard, why shouldn't we be allowed too. Well, now you can.

Maintaining ketosis is now easier than ever with more and more resources becoming readily available. The recipes compiled within this book will explore various yummy low-carb bread loafs, muffins, cookies, burger buns, pizza crusts and so much more!

No more avoiding those delicious foods you love, with just a few humble substitutions and a little self-control, you will be enjoying all of your favorite treats in no time.

Enough about that, let's get to it!

KETO DIET & KETO BREADS

The revolutionary ketogenic diet has been around for many decades, originating in the early 1900's as a treatment for epilepsy. Since then many have adapted this exciting new approach to assist in promoting a healthier lifestyle by adapting a low-carbohydrate, high-fat diet.

Breads form a very fundamental part of our everyday diet and are typically a food you should avoid while eating keto. Everyday breads are easily available in all supermarkets, bakeries, and pastry shops. However, they are a strict no-go while following a keto diet due to the usage of processed ingredients and high carbohydrate value which we will further explore later on.

The world of keto breads is not only restricted to bread loaves. It is expanded to serve you with a variety of breads (dinner rolls, buns, muffins, bagels, pizza crusts, cakes and so on) to make your keto diet journey exciting and full of vibrant flavors.

Why Homemade Keto Bread?

Making keto friendly breads at home is not a difficult task. With the right guidance and willingness, you can easily learn to bake numerous lip-smacking recipes that won't break you out of ketosis. Don't tempt yourself with high carbohydrate bread loaves when you can bake a fresh, healthy, low-carbohydrate, high-fat keto bread alternative within the comfort of your own home.

Compared to unhealthy commercial breads, homemade keto breads are low in bad carbohydrates, high in healthy fats, and protein rich, thanks to its carefully selected keto-friendly ingredients. Commercial breads are also high with added preservatives, additives, and processed ingredients, which in general is a healthy choice to avoid.

One great advantage of homemade breads is that you have total control over all ingredients, you can

be sure to include all quality and fresh ingredients for your keto breads without the need to add any preservatives, artificial colors, or additives.

Due to low carbohydrate values, and lack of any processed wheat based ingredients, ketogenic breads offer countless health advantages. Replacing everyday breads with healthy keto bread options help to:

- Provide an energy boost and increase energy levels throughout the day.
- Maintain a healthy blood sugar level and reduce blood sugar spikes.
- Improve heart health by reducing bad cholesterol level and preventing high blood pressure. It also increases the level of good cholesterol count in the blood.
- Promote natural weight loss and prevent unexpected weight gain.
- Reduce food cravings and thus, minimizes overall food consumption.
- Encourage improved mental health and clarity. (One of my absolute favorites!)

So, What Actually Is The Ketogenic Diet?

The Ketogenic diet is aimed at promoting healthy weight loss and improving holistic health by minimizing the consumption of bad carbohydrates and increasing the consumption of healthy fats. Our body is biologically practiced into relying on carbohydrates as a primary energy source. Stored carbohydrates get converted into glucose within the body in order to fulfil energy requirements to carry out hundreds of everyday tasks.

The Ketogenic diet aims at creating a carbohydrate deficit within the body and increasing the supply of healthy fats; the aim is to convert carbohydrates as our body's primary energy source to healthy fats being the source of fuel. The Keto diet emphasizes consuming meals in a targeted nutrient ratio of fats, carbohydrates and protein. An overall textbook keto diet ratio is divided into the following nutrient proportions:

- 70-75% healthy fats
- 15-20% protein
- 5% carbohydrates

A perfect keto ratio is challenging to achieve for some recipes. The aim is to bake with the most favorable ingredients to give you the best opportunity to fulfil your daily goals without overly compromising on taste and flavor.

A State of Ketosis

When we supply our body with high-fat, low-carbohydrate foods, it creates a deficit of carbohydrates. In such a depleted state, our body explores alternative sources of energy to carry out hundreds of routine bodily functions. Gradually, our body stops relying on carbohydrates for energy requirements and starts replacing its primary energy source with fats as fuel.

In such a state, our body starts producing ketones, which are then used to fulfil energy requirements; this bodily state is known as "ketosis". Ketosis is what promotes healthy weight loss and blesses us with many more health benefits as previously mentioned.

Foods to Avoid

High carbohydrate ingredients are avoided in a ketogenic diet such as starchy vegetables, wheat, rice, pasta, processed bakery products (cake, muffins, etc.), all commercially processed products (fruit juices, sweetened beverages, fried foods, snacks, chips, etc.), beans, and legumes.

Keto Foods

Ingredients rich in healthy fats and moderate in protein values are favored in keto diets and keto breads such as eggs, avocado, butter, coconut oil, olive oil, sesame oil, full fat dairy products (cheese, sour cream, cream cheese etc.), all types of nuts (cashews, walnuts, almonds etc.), bacon, coconut, green vegetables, herbs and spices.

Fruits in Keto Breads

Most fruits contain moderate to high amounts of carbohydrates and for that the reason they are not a preferable choice to add to ketogenic diet recipes. Few exceptions in fruits include several berry options, tomatoes, avocado and olives. Although, berries are allowed in the keto diet, their consumption should be in moderation. Fruits in general should be added with caution in smaller portions to avoid excess carbohydrate intake.

Essential Keto Bread Ingredients

Almond Flour

Almond flour is frequently used in keto breads as a popular low carb flour option. It provides a fine grainy texture to supplement all-purpose flour. Rich in minerals and vitamins, almond flour is prepared from blanched almonds, offering a delicious nutty flavor and does not contain almond skin. Since it can go "bad" fast, it is advised to store it in the fridge or freezer and use as required to help it keep longer.

Coconut Flour

Coconut flour, another great option that is high in healthy fats; an ideal grain-free flour substitution. However, it absorbs a lot of liquid and demands more moisture when baking.

Sesame Flour

Sesame flour is used in a few keto bread recipes and carries its unique flavor. You need to just add the appropriate amount to any bread recipe and make certain to give it a gentle stir to nicely combine all the ingredients.

Flax Meal

Flax meal is prepared from ground flax seeds or linseeds. Flax whole seeds need to be ground into meal in order to obtain a fine texture. It is a great source of vitamin B1, Copper, and Omega-3.

Flax meal is another great replacement for wheat flour in many bread recipes. It can also replace the purpose of eggs as it helps bind together ingredients. If you do not wish to use eggs, replace each egg with a mixture of one Tablespoon ground flax meal in conjunction with three Tablespoons of water.

Almond Meal

Almond meal is not too dissimilar to almond flour. However, it is typically produced from raw (skinned) almonds and holds a slightly coarser texture.

Yeast

Yeast is commonly used as a leavening agent. In bread mixture, added yeast converts the fermentable food sugars into the gas; carbon dioxide. This gas causes the mixture to expand or rise and form air pockets or bubbles.

Eggs

It is recommended to keep eggs at room temperature before adding to recipes. Eggs ensure tender crust and add a generous protein boost to bread recipes.

Coconut/Olive Oil & Butter

Many bread recipes include a stable oil in order to combine all ingredients together to maintain an ideal consistency. Oil helps to withstand high oven temperatures and ensures a smooth bread texture. Coconut, olive or sesame oil is a great substitute for regular oils as they are high with healthy fats and low in cholesterol. Butter along with added oil helps in providing the brown texture to bread crust.

Cream of Tartar

Cream of tartar is also referred as Potassium Bitartrate. It is a byproduct of wine preparation. Adding cream of tartar to egg whites strengthens its overall stability. It helps to maintain fluffy texture of a whisked mixture.

Xanthan Gum

Xanthan Gum is used in a powder form as a thickener and stabilizer. It is gluten free and contains no carbohydrates. Used in small quantity, it helps to achieve perfectly textured breads.

Low Carb Sweeteners

Stevia, Splenda, honey, and coconut sugar are popular low carbohydrate sweeteners used in keto bread as a sugar replacement. They contain minimal to no-amount of carbohydrates, making them an ideal replacement for sugar in keto breads. Due to low sugar levels, they prevent blood sugar spikes and enable natural weight loss.

- Stevia is a herb; stevia sweetener contains no calories, vitamins or any other nutrients. Liquid stevia drops are commonly used, however, its granular form is also used in many bread recipes.
- Coconut sugar is a natural sugar. This low carb sweetener is prepared from sugary circulating fluid of the coconut plant. Coconut sugar is less frequently used in comparison with other sweeteners.
- Erythritol is a low-carb sweetener, just like Stevia. It is a form of sugar alcohol that is used to add sweetness to different types of bread recipes without increasing total carbohydrate value.

How To Make Perfect Keto Breads

- Sifting is a process that removes lumps in the flour. It provides required oxygen to ingredients to aerate the bread batter. Sifted flour is much lighter than unsifted flour. Unsifted flour becomes compressed and heavy. However, after sifting, it gains a nice consistency throughout. Not all recipes use sifted flour, but you can quite easily replace them with a sifted variety if you please.
- A silicon pan is not advised to use for baking keto breads, as it prevents breads from rising properly. It is advised to use a proper firm baking or loaf pans for an even heat distribution and to allow the bread to correctly rise.
- Generally, you do not want to over mix a dough mixture. It creates a hollow crust as the dough will instantly deflate. Only mix the ingredients until they form an consistent texture. Although not required for all bread recipes, if time permits, allow the dough to rest for at least 30 minutes before putting it in the oven.
- In many cases, the baking paper may end up sticking to the bread. Allow the bread to cool down completely, and then remove the baking paper. Alternatively, put a wet towel over the paper to soften it a little and then remove it.
- Once the baking time has concluded, place the bread onto a cooling rack. It ensures that the bread doesn't become moist; also it allows the bread to slowly firm up, making it easy to slice.

CHAPTER 1
KETO BREAD LOAFS

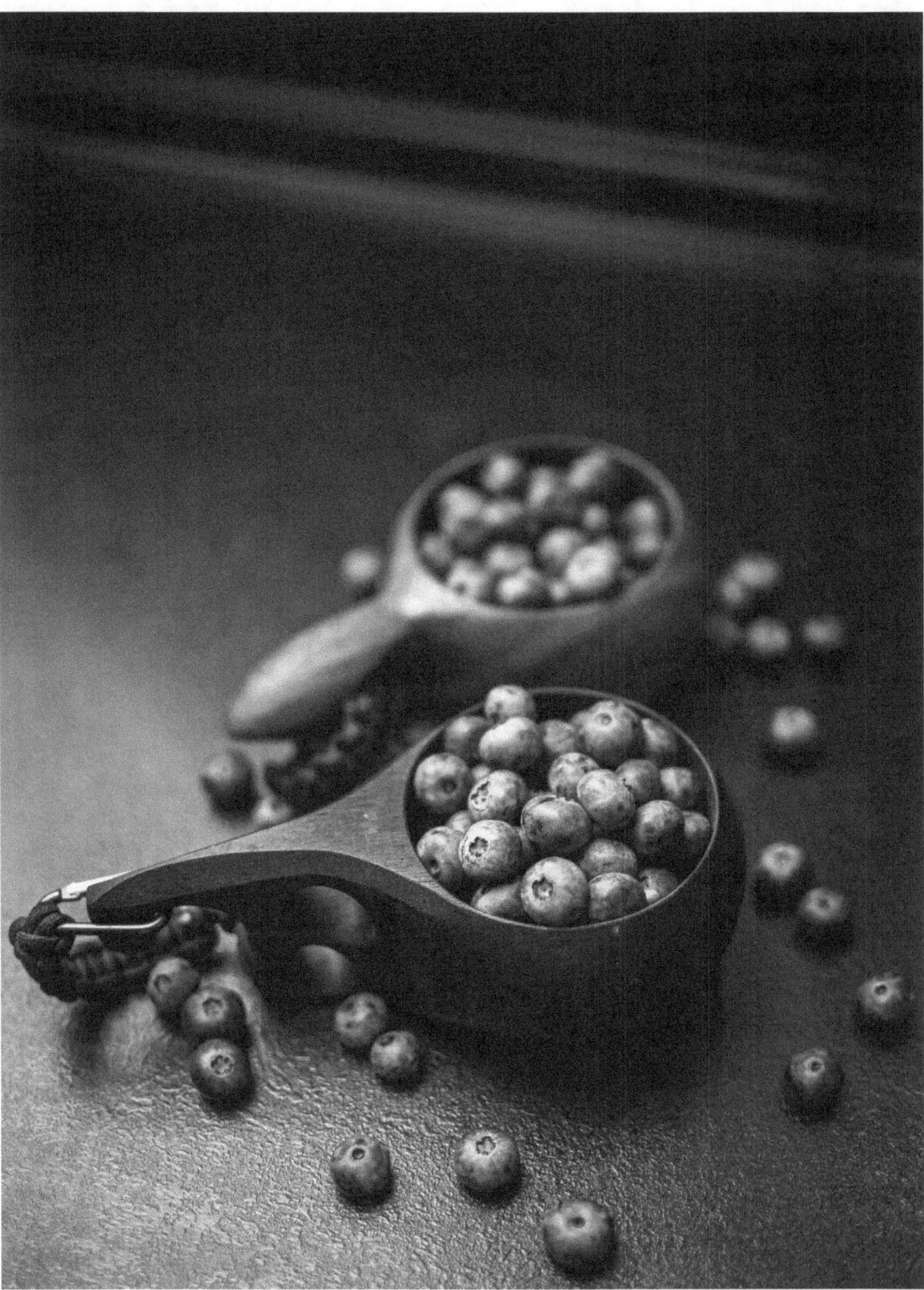

Keto Blueberry Bread

Servings:
10-12

Preparation Time:
65-70 mins

Method:
Bake

INGREDIENTS:

5 eggs, lightly beaten

2 teaspoons baking powder

¼ cup almond flour

½ cup blueberries

½ teaspoon salt

½ cup almond butter, melted

½ cup almond milk, unsweetened

¼ cup ghee

DIRECTIONS:

1. Preheat an oven to 350°F-176°C. Prepare a medium-size bread pan or loaf pan by lining it with a parchment paper. Grease it with some coconut oil or butter. (You can also use coconut oil cooking spray to grease)
2. Combine the almond flour, baking powder, and salt in mixing bowl and mix well.
3. Add the almond butter and ghee; combine well until there is no lumps.
4. Whisk the eggs and milk in another bowl, mix in the blueberries.
5. Combine both mixtures with each other. Combine well until smooth batter is formed without any visible lumps.
6. Take the prepared batter and slowly pour it in the greased bread or loaf pan; mounding batter slightly in the center so that it creates a rounded top.
7. Place the bread or loaf pan in the preheated oven and bake for 45 minutes or until turns golden brown. You can check by inserting a toothpick; when the bread is baked well, toothpick comes out clean.
8. Take out the bread pan and allow it to cool down on a wired rack for at least 10-20 minutes. Shake the pan gently and take out the bread from the pan.
9. Cut into slices and serve!

NUTRITIONAL VALUES (PER SERVING):

Calories:146
F:13g C:4g fi:1g P:5g

Basic Keto Bread

Servings:
10-12

Preparation Time:
80-90 mins

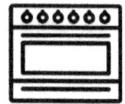

Method:
Bake

INGREDIENTS:

¼ cup coconut flour

1 cup almond flour

¼ teaspoon salt

¼ teaspoons baking powder

½ teaspoon arrowroot powder

⅓ cup butter (melted)

1 Tablespoon active dry yeast

½ teaspoon cream of tartar

12 egg whites

10-15 drops liquid Stevia

DIRECTIONS:

1. Preheat an oven to 325°F-162°C. Prepare a medium-size bread pan or loaf pan by lining it with a parchment paper.
2. In a blender or food processor, blend the almond flour, coconut flour, baking powder, arrowroot powder, and salt until thoroughly combined. Add the butter and blend until turn crumbly.
3. Add the yeast and pulse until combined.
4. In a mixing bowl, add the cream of tartar over egg whites and beat well until stiff peaks form.
5. Combine both the mixtures. Combine well until smooth batter is formed without any visible lumps.
6. Take the prepared batter and slowly pour it in the greased bread or loaf pan; mounding batter slightly in the center so that it creates a rounded top.
7. Place the bread or loaf pan in the preheated oven and bake for 40 minutes or until turns golden brown. You can check by inserting a toothpick; when the bread is baked well, toothpick comes out clean.
8. Take out the bread pan and allow it to cool down on a wired rack for at least 10-20 minutes. Shake the pan gently and take out the bread from the pan.
9. Cut into slices and serve!

NUTRITIONAL VALUES (PER SERVING):

Calories:246
F:24g C:5g fi:3g P:9g

Classic Coconut Bread

Servings:
4-6

Preparation Time:
55-65 mins

Method:
Bake

INGREDIENTS:

- ½ cup coconut flour
- 6 eggs (lightly beaten)
- ½ cup butter (melted)
- 1 teaspoon baking powder
- ¼ teaspoon salt

DIRECTIONS:

1. Preheat an oven to 350°F-176°C. Prepare a medium-size bread pan or loaf pan by greasing it with some coconut oil or butter. (You can also use coconut oil cooking spray to grease).
2. In a mixing bowl, mix the coconut flour, baking powder, and salt until thoroughly combined.
3. In a large bowl, beat the eggs until turn frothy. Add the butter and beat until thoroughly combined.
4. Combine both mixtures with each other. Combine well until smooth batter is formed without any visible lumps.
5. Take the prepared batter and slowly pour it in the greased bread or loaf pan; mounding batter slightly in the center so that it creates a rounded top.
6. Place the bread or loaf pan in the preheated oven and bake for 45 minutes or until turns golden brown. You can check by inserting a toothpick; when the bread is baked well, toothpick comes out clean.
7. Take out the bread pan and allow it to cool down on a wired rack for at least 10-20 minutes. Shake the pan gently and take out the bread from the pan.
8. Cut into slices and serve!

NUTRITIONAL VALUES (PER SERVING):

Calories:126
F:11g C:4g Fi:0.5g P:5g

Classic Keto Bread

Servings:
6-8

Preparation Time:
40-45 mins

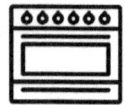

Method:
Bake

INGREDIENTS:

- 6 large eggs, whites and yolk separated
- 1 ½ cups almond flour
- ¼ teaspoon cream of tartar
- 1 pinch salt
- 4 Tablespoons butter (melted)
- 3 teaspoons baking powder

DIRECTIONS:

1. Preheat an oven to 375°F-190°C. Prepare a medium-size bread pan or loaf pan by greasing it with some coconut oil or butter. (You can also use coconut oil cooking spray to grease)
2. In a bowl, beat the egg whites and cream of tartar.
3. In a blender, blend the egg yolks, 1/3 egg whites, almond flour, butter, baking powder and salt.
4. Add remaining 2/3 egg whites and blend again.
5. Take the prepared batter and slowly pour it in the greased bread or loaf pan; mounding batter slightly in the center so that it creates a rounded top.
6. Place the bread or loaf pan in the preheated oven and bake for 30 minutes or until turns golden brown. You can check by inserting a toothpick; when the bread is baked well, toothpick comes out clean.
7. Take out the bread pan and allow it to cool down on a wired rack for at least 10-20 minutes. Shake the pan gently and take out the bread from the pan.
8. Cut into slices and serve!

NUTRITIONAL VALUES (PER SERVING):

Calories:246
F:24g C:5g fi:3g P:9g

Mix Seed Almond Bread

Servings:
18-20

Preparation Time:
60-70 mins

Method:
Bake

INGREDIENTS:

1 ½ cup almond flour
½ teaspoon salt
1 cup pumpkin seeds
1 cup sunflower seeds
½ cup chia seeds
2 Tablespoons olive oil
1 cup sesame seeds
5 eggs

DIRECTIONS:

1. Preheat an oven to 350°F-176°C. Prepare a medium-size bread pan or loaf pan by lining it with a parchment paper.
2. Add the almond flour and the eggs in a blender or food processor and blend once.
3. Add the seeds, olive oil, and salt; blende the mixture again the seeds are ground. Do not over blend.
4. Take the prepared batter and slowly pour it in the greased bread or loaf pan; mounding batter slightly in the center so that it creates a rounded top.
5. Place the bread or loaf pan in the preheated oven and bake for 50 minutes or until turns golden brown. You can check by inserting a toothpick; when the bread is baked well, toothpick comes out clean.
6. Take out the bread pan and allow it to cool down on a wired rack for at least 10-20 minutes. Shake the pan gently and take out the bread from the pan.
7. Cut into slices and serve!

NUTRITIONAL VALUES (PER SERVING):

Calories:162
F:13g C:3g fi:1g P:6g

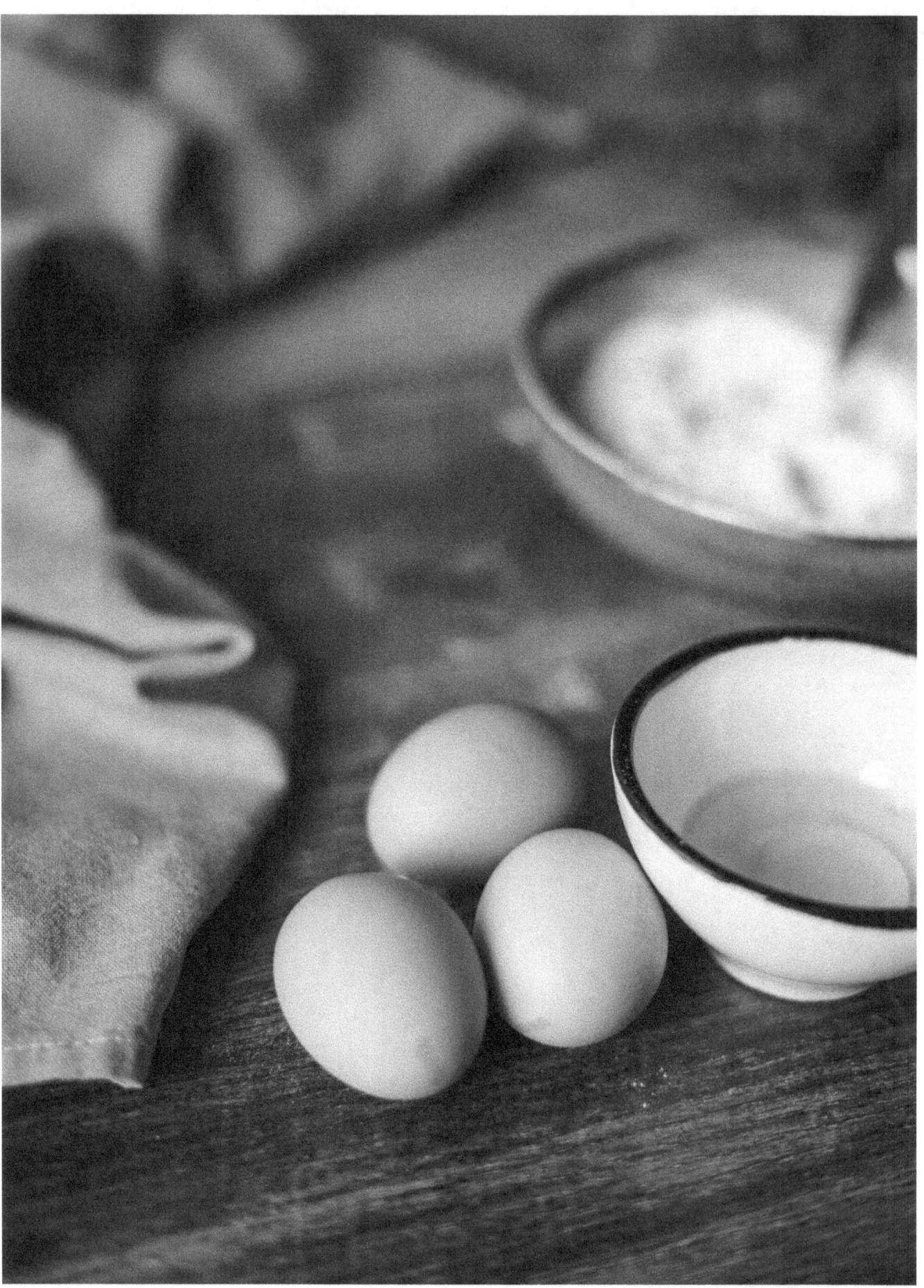

Perky Pumpkin Bread

Servings:
10-12

Preparation Time:
70-80 mins

Method:
Bake

INGREDIENTS:

- 2 cups almond flour
- ¼ cup pumpkin seeds
- ½ cup coconut flour sifted
- 4 eggs lightly beaten
- ⅓ cup butter, melted
- ¾ cup Erythritol
- 2 teaspoons pumpkin pie spice
- ¾ cup pumpkin puree
- 2 teaspoons baking powder
- ¼ teaspoon sea salt

DIRECTIONS:

1. Preheat an oven to 375°F-190°C. Prepare a medium-size bread pan or loaf pan by lining it with a parchment paper. Grease it with some coconut oil or butter. (You can also use coconut oil cooking spray to grease)
2. In a mixing bowl and combine the baking powder, almond flour, pumpkin pie spice, salt, and erythritol. Mix in the pumpkin puree and butter.
3. Add one egg at a time; whisk the mixture well.
4. Take the prepared batter and slowly pour it in the greased bread or loaf pan; mounding batter slightly in the center so that it creates a rounded top. Top it with some pumpkin seeds.
5. Place the bread or loaf pan in the preheated oven and bake for 50 minutes or until turns golden brown. You can check by inserting a toothpick; when the bread is baked well, toothpick comes out clean.
6. Take out the bread pan and allow it to cool down on a wired rack for at least 10-20 minutes. Shake the pan gently and take out the bread from the pan.
7. Cut into slices and serve!

NUTRITIONAL VALUES (PER SERVING):

Calories: 214
F:18g C:4g fi1g P:8g

Keto Cornbread

Servings:
4-6

Preparation Time:
60-70 mins

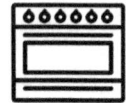
Method:
Bake

INGREDIENTS:

½ cup coconut flour

¼ cup coconut oil (melted)

2 Tablespoons apple cider vinegar

4 eggs

1 cup water

½ teaspoon baking soda

½ teaspoon garlic powder

¼ teaspoon sea salt

DIRECTIONS:

1. Preheat an oven to 350°F-176°C. Prepare a medium-size bread pan or loaf pan by greasing it with some coconut oil or butter. (You can also use coconut oil cooking spray to grease)
2. Blend the eggs in the blender. Set aside for 20 minutes.
3. Add water, coconut oil and apple cider vinegar in the blender. Blend for about 20-30 seconds.
4. Add the coconut flour, baking soda, garlic powder and salt. Blend for 1 minute.
5. Take the prepared batter and slowly pour it in the greased bread or loaf pan; mounding batter slightly in the center so that it creates a rounded top.
6. Place the bread or loaf pan in the preheated oven and bake for 45 minutes or until turns golden brown. You can check by inserting a toothpick; when the bread is baked well, toothpick comes out clean.
7. Take out the bread pan and allow it to cool down on a wired rack for at least 10-20 minutes. Shake the pan gently and take out the bread from the pan.
8. Cut into slices and serve!

NUTRITIONAL VALUES (PER SERVING):

Calories:103
F:7g C:4g Fi:2g P:3g

Yogurt Cinnamon Bread

Servings:
4-6

Preparation Time:
30-40 mins

Method:
Bake

INGREDIENTS:

- 3 Tablespoons butter, melted
- 2 Tablespoons water
- 1 teaspoon cinnamon
- 1 teaspoon vinegar
- 3 eggs
- ½ cup coconut flour
- ⅓ cup Greek yogurt or coconut milk
- ½ teaspoon baking powder
- ½ teaspoon baking soda
- 5 drops liquid Stevia

DIRECTIONS:

1. Preheat an oven to 350°F-176°C. Prepare a medium-size bread pan or loaf pan by lining it with a parchment paper. Grease it with some coconut oil or butter. (You can also use coconut oil cooking spray to grease)
2. Add the coconut flour, cinnamon, baking powder, baking soda and Stevia in the blender. Blend well.
3. Add the yogurt, butter, water and vinegar in the blender. Blend to combine well.
4. Take the prepared batter and slowly pour it in the greased bread or loaf pan; mounding batter slightly in the center so that it creates a rounded top.
5. Place the bread or loaf pan in the preheated oven and bake for 30 minutes or until turns golden brown. You can check by inserting a toothpick; when the bread is baked well, toothpick comes out clean.
6. Take out the bread pan and allow it to cool down on a wired rack for at least 10-20 minutes. Shake the pan gently and take out the bread from the pan.
7. Cut into slices and serve!

NUTRITIONAL VALUES (PER SERVING):

Calories:146
F:9g C:4g Fi:1g P:6g

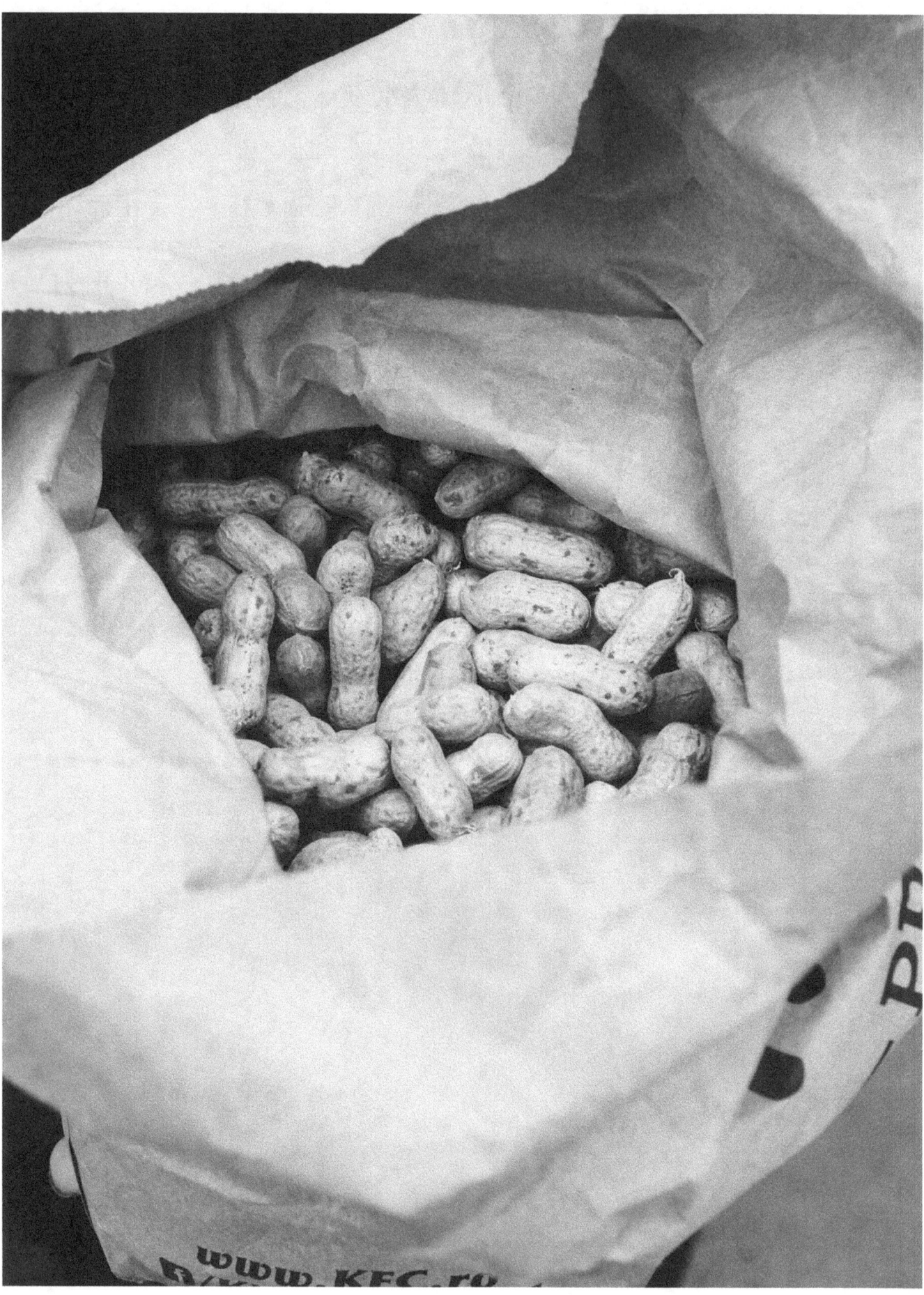

Keto Peanut Butter Bread

Servings:
4-5

Preparation Time:
25-30 mins

Method:
Bake

INGREDIENTS:

3 large eggs

5 drops liquid Stevia

1 Tablespoon cider vinegar

½ teaspoon baking soda

16 Tablespoons peanut butter, unsweetened

A dash salt

DIRECTIONS:

1. Preheat an oven to 350°F-176°C. Grease two 3"x5" mini loaf pans with some coconut oil or butter. (You can also use coconut oil cooking spray to grease)
2. In a mixing bowl, combine all the ingredients. Combine well until smooth batter is formed.
3. Take the prepared batter and slowly pour it in the greased loaf pans; mounding batter slightly in the center so that it creates a rounded top.
4. Place the loaf pans in the preheated oven and bake for 25 minutes or until turns golden brown. You can check by inserting a toothpick; when the bread is baked well, toothpick comes out clean.
5. Take out the bread pan and allow it to cool down on a wired rack for at least 10-20 minutes. Shake the pan gently and take out the bread from the pan.
6. Cut into slices and serve!

NUTRITIONAL VALUES (PER SERVING):

Calories:142
F:13g C:3g Fi:0g P:8g

Super Cheese Bread

Servings:
12-14

Preparation Time:
40-50 mins

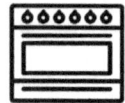

Method:
Bake

INGREDIENTS:

- ½ cup mozzarella cheese, shredded
- ¼ cup coconut flour
- 3 Tablespoons water
- 5 ounces of cream cheese
- 3 eggs
- ¼ cup butter
- ½ teaspoon sea salt
- 2 teaspoon baking powder
- ⅔ cup almond flour
- ½ cup parmesan cheese, finely shredded
- ½ teaspoon sea salt

DIRECTIONS:

1. Preheat an oven to 400°F-204°C. Prepare a medium-size bread pan or loaf pan by greasing it with some coconut oil or butter. (You can also use coconut oil cooking spray to grease)
2. In a mixing bowl, add the cream cheese and butter. Whisk the mixture, stir in the remaining ingredients. Combine well until smooth batter is formed without any visible lumps.
3. Take the prepared batter and slowly pour it in the greased bread or loaf pan; mounding batter slightly in the center so that it creates a rounded top.
4. Place the bread or loaf pan in the preheated oven and bake for 30 minutes or until turns golden brown. You can check by inserting a toothpick; when the bread is baked well, toothpick comes out clean.
5. Take out the bread pan and allow it to cool down on a wired rack for at least 10-20 minutes. Shake the pan gently and take out the bread from the pan.
6. Cut into slices and serve!

NUTRITIONAL VALUES (PER SERVING):

Calories:134
F:8g C:2g Fi:0g P:5g

Almond Cream Bread

Servings:
7-8

Preparation Time:
45-50 mins

Method:
Bake

INGREDIENTS:

4 large eggs

1 cup almond flour

¼ cup sesame seeds flour

1 Tablespoon sesame seeds

2 Tablespoons psyllium husk powder

1 cup cream cheese

4 Tablespoons sesame seeds oil or olive oil

1 teaspoon salt

1 teaspoon baking soda

Egg wash (1 egg yolk combined with 1 Tablespoon coconut oil)

DIRECTIONS:

1. Preheat an oven to 400°F-204°C. Prepare a baking sheet by lining it with a parchment paper. Grease it with some coconut oil or butter. (You can also use coconut oil cooking spray to grease)
2. Beat the eggs in a mixing bowl, until turn fluffy. Mix in the cream cheese and sesame seeds oil; combine well.
3. Add the almond flour, sesame seeds flour, psyllium husk powder, salt, and baking soda. Combine well.
4. Place the dough over the lined baking sheet; give it a loaf shape.
5. Beat the egg yolks and coconut oil in a bowl. Brush the loaf with egg wash and sprinkle with sesame seeds.
6. Bake for 30 minutes or until turns golden brown.
7. Take out the baking sheet and allow it to cool down on a wired rack for at least 10-20 minutes.
8. Serve and enjoy!

NUTRITIONAL VALUES (PER SERVING):

Calories: 224
F: 24g C: 5g Fi: 1g P: 7g

Peanut Cream Bread

Servings:
4-5

Preparation Time:
55-60 mins

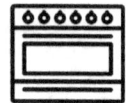

Method:
Bake

INGREDIENTS:

- ¾ cup peanut flour
- 1 ½ teaspoons baking powder
- ¼ teaspoon salt
- 8 ounces of cream cheese (softened)
- 6 eggs yolks
- 6 Tablespoons butter (melted)
- 1 ½ teaspoons vanilla extract
- 15-20 drops liquid Stevia

DIRECTIONS:

1. Preheat an oven to 350°F-176°C. Prepare a medium-size bread pan or loaf pan by greasing it with some coconut oil or butter. (You can also use coconut oil cooking spray to grease)
2. In a mixing bowl, whisk the peanut flour, baking powder, and salt until thoroughly combined.
3. In another bowl, mix the cream cheese and butter. Add the egg yolks, sweetener and vanilla extract and mix until thoroughly combined.
4. Combine both mixtures with each other. Combine well until smooth batter is formed without any visible lumps.
5. Take the prepared batter and slowly pour it in the greased bread or loaf pan; mounding batter slightly in the center so that it creates a rounded top.
6. Place the bread or loaf pan in the preheated oven and bake for 25 minutes or until turns golden brown. You can check by inserting a toothpick; when the bread is baked well, toothpick comes out clean.
7. Take out the bread pan and allow it to cool down on a wired rack for at least 10-20 minutes. Shake the pan gently and take out the bread from the pan.
8. Cut into slices and serve!

NUTRITIONAL VALUES (PER SERVING):

Calories: 242
F:18g C:6g Fi:3g P:14g

Caraway Coconut Bread

Servings:
14-16

Preparation Time:
70 mins

Method:
Bake

INGREDIENTS:

Dry ingredients:

2 Tablespoons caraway seeds

1 Tablespoon + 1 teaspoon baking powder

2 cups flaxseed (ground)

1 cup coconut flour

1 Tablespoon Erythritol

¼ cup chia seeds (ground)

1 teaspoon salt

Wet ingredients:

8 eggs, whites and yolk separated

1 cup water, warm

½ cup ghee

⅓ cup apple cider vinegar

2 Tablespoons sesame oil

DIRECTIONS:

1. Preheat an oven to 350°F-176°C. Prepare a medium-size bread pan or loaf pan by greasing it with some coconut oil or butter. (You can also use coconut oil cooking spray to grease)
2. Add the dry ingredients in a bowl. Mix thoroughly.
3. Beat the egg whites and set aside. In another bowl, whisk the yolk; mix in the ghee and sesame oil.
4. Add the dry mixture to the egg yolk mixture. Mix thoroughly. Add the vinegar and water and mix again. Add egg whites and continue mixing.
5. Take the prepared batter and slowly pour it in the greased bread or loaf pan; mounding batter slightly in the center so that it creates a rounded top.
6. Place the bread or loaf pan in the preheated oven and bake for 60 minutes or until turns golden brown. You can check by inserting a toothpick; when the bread is baked well, toothpick comes out clean.
7. Take out the bread pan and allow it to cool down on a wired rack for at least 10-20 minutes. Shake the pan gently and take out the bread from the pan.
8. Cut into slices and serve!

NUTRITIONAL VALUES (PER SERVING):

Calories: 246
F:21g C:9g fi:4g P:8g

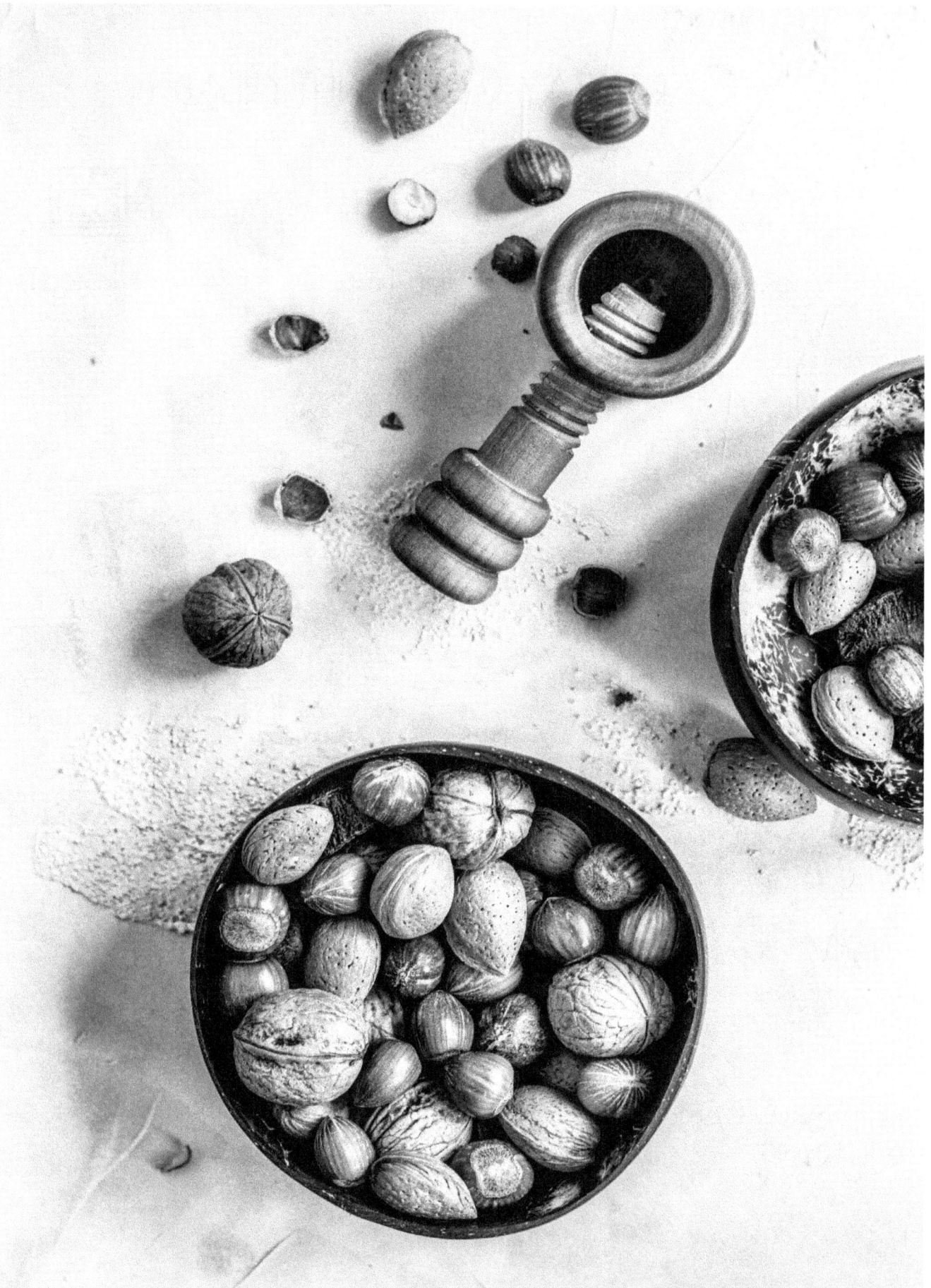

Wonder Walnut Bread

Servings:
10-12

Preparation Time:
70-80 mins

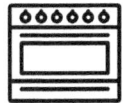

Method:
Bake

INGREDIENTS:

- 2 cups almond flour
- ½ cup coconut flour
- 1 cup butter (melted)
- 4 egg (lightly beaten)
- 1 teaspoon ground cinnamon
- ½ teaspoon ground nutmeg
- ¼ teaspoon ground ginger
- 1 ½ teaspoon baking powder
- ¼ teaspoon salt
- 1 teaspoon liquid Stevia
- ⅓ cup heavy cream
- 1 teaspoon vanilla extract
- ½ cup chopped walnuts

DIRECTIONS:

1. Preheat an oven to 350°F-176°C. Prepare a medium-size bread pan or loaf pan by greasing it with some coconut oil or butter. (You can also use coconut oil cooking spray to grease)
2. In a mixing bowl, whisk the almond flour, coconut flour, baking powder, cinnamon, nutmeg, ginger, and salt.
3. In another bowl, whisk the butter, egg, sweetener, heavy cream, and vanilla extract until thoroughly combined.
4. Combine both mixtures with each other. Add the walnuts; combine well until smooth batter is formed without any visible lumps.
5. Take the prepared batter and slowly pour it in the greased bread or loaf pan; mounding batter slightly in the center so that it creates a rounded top.
6. Place the bread or loaf pan in the preheated oven and bake for 50-60 minutes or until turns golden brown. You can check by inserting a toothpick; when the bread is baked well, toothpick comes out clean.
7. Take out the bread pan and allow it to cool down on a wired rack for at least 10-20 minutes. Shake the pan gently and take out the bread from the pan.
8. Cut into slices and serve!

NUTRITIONAL VALUES (PER SERVING):

Calories:192
F:22g C:6g fi:2g P:5g

Poppy Seed Bread

Servings:
8-10

Preparation Time:
70-80 mins

Method:
Bake

INGREDIENTS:

3 cups almond flour

3 Tablespoons poppy seeds

2 teaspoon baking powder

¼ eggs (lightly beaten)

1 teaspoon liquid Stevia

4 Tablespoons butter (melted)

⅓ cup unsweetened almond milk

Zest and juice from 1 lemon

DIRECTIONS:

1. Preheat an oven to 325°F-162°C. Prepare a medium-size bread pan or loaf pan by greasing it with some coconut oil or butter. (You can also use coconut oil cooking spray to grease)
2. In a mixing bowl, whisk the almond flour, poppy seeds, baking powder, and salt.
3. In another mixing bowl, whisk the eggs, sweetener, butter, almond milk, lemon zest, and lemon juice until thoroughly combined.
4. Combine both mixtures with each other.
5. Combine well until smooth batter is formed without any visible lumps.
6. Take the prepared batter and slowly pour it in the greased bread or loaf pan; mounding batter slightly in the center so that it creates a rounded top.
7. Place the bread or loaf pan in the preheated oven and bake for 50-60 minutes or until turns golden brown. You can check by inserting a toothpick; when the bread is baked well, toothpick comes out clean.
8. Take out the bread pan and allow it to cool down on a wired rack for at least 10-20 minutes. Shake the pan gently and take out the bread from the pan.
9. Cut into slices and serve!

NUTRITIONAL VALUES (PER SERVING):

Calories:143
F:12g C:3g Fi:0g P:14g

Keto Round Bread

Servings:
6

Preparation Time:
20-30 mins

Method:
Bake

INGREDIENTS:

- ⅔ cups almond flour
- 3 eggs
- ½ teaspoon salt
- ½ teaspoon baking powder
- 4 Tablespoons olive oil
- 2 teaspoons xylitol or 5 drops liquid Stevia

DIRECTIONS:

1. Preheat an oven to 350°F-176°C. Prepare a baking sheet by lining it with a parchment paper. Grease it with some coconut oil or butter. (You can also use coconut oil cooking spray to grease)
2. Beat 1 egg white in mixing a bowl until turns stiff.
3. In another bowl, mix other ingredients and mix in the egg white. Whisk the mixture gently.
4. Drop a Tablespoon over the greases sheet and spread to make a circles but not too thin circle. Repeat until you finish the batter; you should get 6 rounds.
5. Bake for until turns golden brown.
6. Take out the baking sheet and allow it to cool down on a wired rack for at least 10-20 minutes.
7. Serve and enjoy!

NUTRITIONAL VALUES (PER SERVING):

Calories:201
F:21g C:4g Fi:1g P:6g

Almond Olive Bread

Servings:
10-12

Preparation Time:
70-80 mins

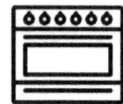
Method:
Bake

INGREDIENTS:

½ cup + 2 Tablespoons olive oil

¼ cup almond milk

3 eggs

3 cups almond flour

2 teaspoons baking powder

1 teaspoon baking soda

¼ teaspoon salt coconut flour

1 cup almond flour

¼ teaspoon salt

DIRECTIONS:

1. Preheat an oven to 300°F-148°C. Prepare a medium-size bread pan or loaf pan by greasing it with some coconut oil or butter. (You can also use coconut oil cooking spray to grease)
2. Add the wet ingredients in a bowl. Whisk thoroughly.
3. In another bowl, mix all the dry ingredients.
4. Combine both mixtures with each other. Combine well until smooth batter is formed without any visible lumps.
5. Take the prepared batter and slowly pour it in the greased bread or loaf pan; mounding batter slightly in the center so that it creates a rounded top.
6. Place the bread or loaf pan in the preheated oven and bake for 55-60 minutes or until turns golden brown. You can check by inserting a toothpick; when the bread is baked well, toothpick comes out clean.
7. Take out the bread pan and allow it to cool down on a wired rack for at least 10-20 minutes. Shake the pan gently and take out the bread from the pan.
8. Cut into slices and serve!

NUTRITIONAL VALUES (PER SERVING):

Calories:368
F:28g C:8g fi:2g P:11g

Keto Flaxseed Bread

Servings:
4-6

Preparation Time:
90 mins

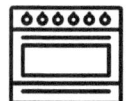

Method:
Bake

INGREDIENTS:

1 teaspoon baking soda

½ teaspoon salt

1 ½ cups almond flour

1/3 cup coconut flour

2 Tablespoons ground flaxseed

10-15 drops liquid Stevia

6 eggs

1 Tablespoon butter (melted)

1 Tablespoon coconut oil

1 teaspoon apple cider vinegar

DIRECTIONS:

1. Preheat an oven to 300°F-148°C. Prepare a medium-size bread pan or loaf pan by greasing it with some coconut oil or butter. (You can also use coconut oil cooking spray to grease)
2. In a mixing bowl, combine the almond flour, coconut flour, flaxseed, sweetener, baking soda, and salt until thoroughly combined.
3. In another bowl, beat the eggs until light and frothy; mix in the butter, coconut oil, and apple cider vinegar.
4. Combine both mixtures with each other. Combine well until smooth batter is formed without any visible lumps.
5. Take the prepared batter and slowly pour it in the greased bread or loaf pan; mounding batter slightly in the center so that it creates a rounded top.
6. Place the bread or loaf pan in the preheated oven and bake for 50-60 minutes or until turns golden brown. You can check by inserting a toothpick; when the bread is baked well, toothpick comes out clean.
7. Take out the bread pan and allow it to cool down on a wired rack for at least 10-20 minutes. Shake the pan gently and take out the bread from the pan.
8. Cut into slices and serve!

NUTRITIONAL VALUES (PER SERVING):

Calories: 208
F:19g C:8g fi:2g P:10g

Coconut Mix Seed Bread

  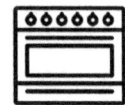

Servings: 4-5

Preparation Time: 55-60 mins

Method: Bake

INGREDIENTS:

½ cup packed ground flaxseed

½ cup coconut flour

10 drops liquid Stevia

¼ teaspoon salt

2 Tablespoons ground chia seeds

1 teaspoon ground anise seeds

½ teaspoon baking soda

4 eggs, white and yolk separated

¼ cup extra virgin olive oil

1 Tablespoon sesame oil

1 teaspoon cream of tartar

½ cup warm water

2 Tablespoons apple cider vinegar

DIRECTIONS:

1. Preheat an oven to 350°F-176°C. Prepare a medium-size bread pan or loaf pan by greasing it with some coconut oil or butter. (You can also use coconut oil cooking spray to grease)
2. In a mixing bowl, mix the flaxseed, coconut flour, chia seeds, anise seeds, baking soda, sweetener and salt until thoroughly combined.
3. In another bowl, whisk the egg yolks, olive oil, and sesame oil until thoroughly combined and set aside.
4. In another bowl, sprinkle cream of tartar over egg whites; whisk until stiff peaks form.
5. Combine both mixtures with each other. Add water and apple cider vinegar and stir until thoroughly combined.
6. Add the egg whites; combine well until smooth batter is formed without any visible lumps.
7. Take the prepared batter and slowly pour it in the greased bread or loaf pan; mounding batter slightly in the center so that it creates a rounded top.
8. Place the bread or loaf pan in the preheated oven and bake for 40 minutes or until turns golden brown. You can check by inserting a toothpick; when the bread is baked well, toothpick comes out clean.
9. Take out the bread pan and allow it to cool down on a wired rack for at least 10-20 minutes. Shake the pan gently and take out the bread from the pan.
10. Cut into slices and serve!

NUTRITIONAL VALUES (PER SERVING):

Calories: 184
F: 14g C: 12g Fi: 2g P: 6g

CHAPTER 2
SPECIAL KETO BREADS

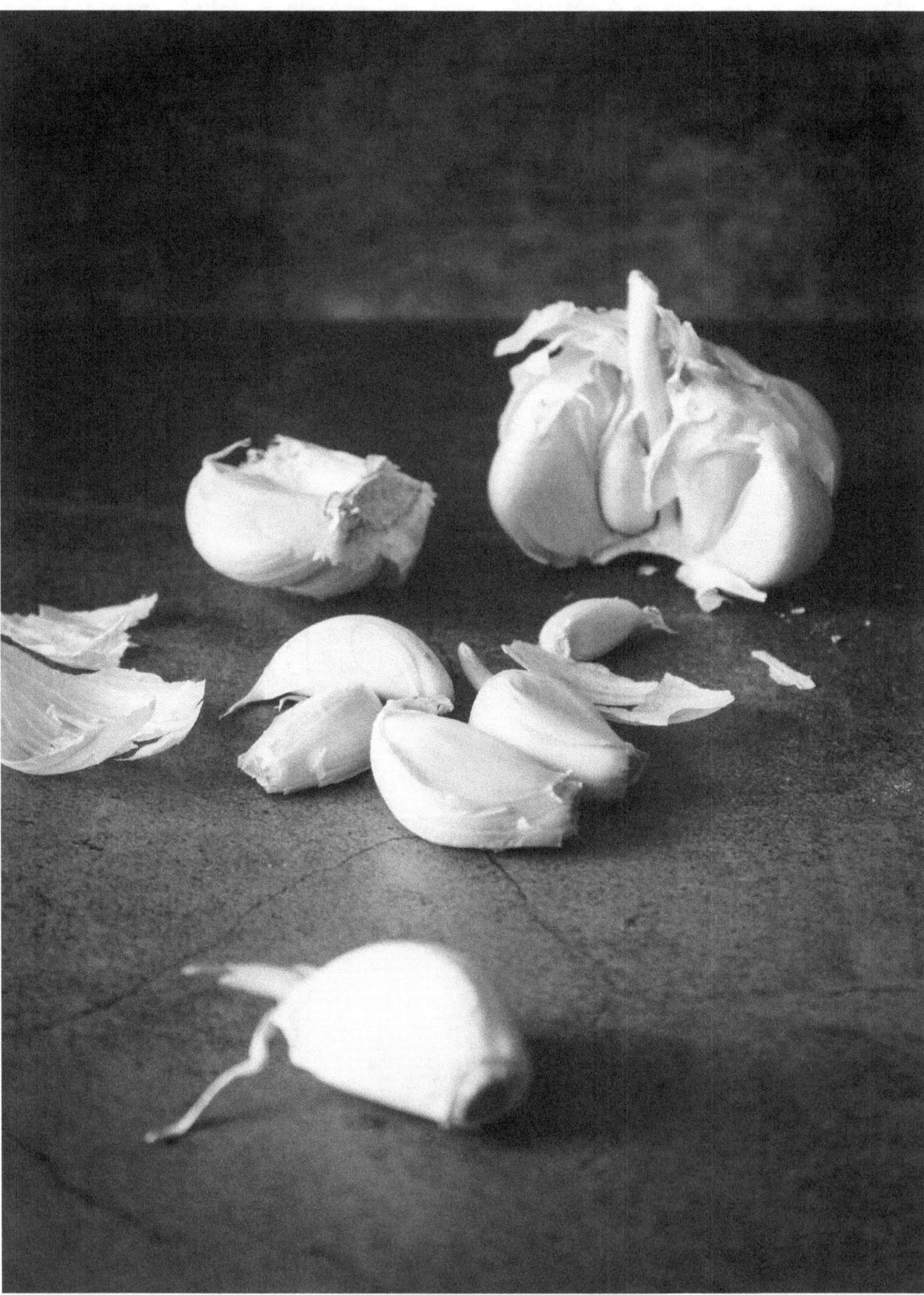

All Time Favorite Garlic Bread

Servings:
6-8

Preparation Time:
30-40 mins

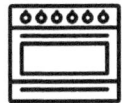

Method:
Bake

INGREDIENTS:

¾ cup almond flour

2 cups shredded mozzarella cheese

2 Tablespoons cream cheese

4 garlic cloves (minced)

1 teaspoon baking powder

1 egg (lightly beaten)

1 Tablespoon butter (melted)

1 Tablespoon chopped fresh basil or parsley leaves

DIRECTIONS:

1. Preheat an oven to 425°F-232°C. Prepare a baking sheet by lining it with a parchment paper. Grease it with some coconut oil or butter. (You can also use coconut oil cooking spray to grease)
2. In a mixing bowl, combine the almond flour, garlic, and baking powder until thoroughly combined.
3. In a microwave, melt 1 1/2 cups mozzarella cheese and cream cheese. Combine well.
4. Add the melted mixture to dry ingredients and stir until combined. Add the egg; combine well until smooth batter is formed without any visible lumps. Shape into oval dough.
5. Place the dough over the lined baking sheet, brush it with the butter and sprinkle remaining 1/2 cup mozzarella cheese and bake for 15 minutes or until turns golden brown.
6. Take out the baking sheet and allow it to cool down on a wired rack for at least 10-20 minutes. Sprinkle with some basil leaves.
7. Serve and enjoy!

NUTRITIONAL VALUES (PER SERVING):

Calories:113
F:9g C:3g fi:0g P:7g

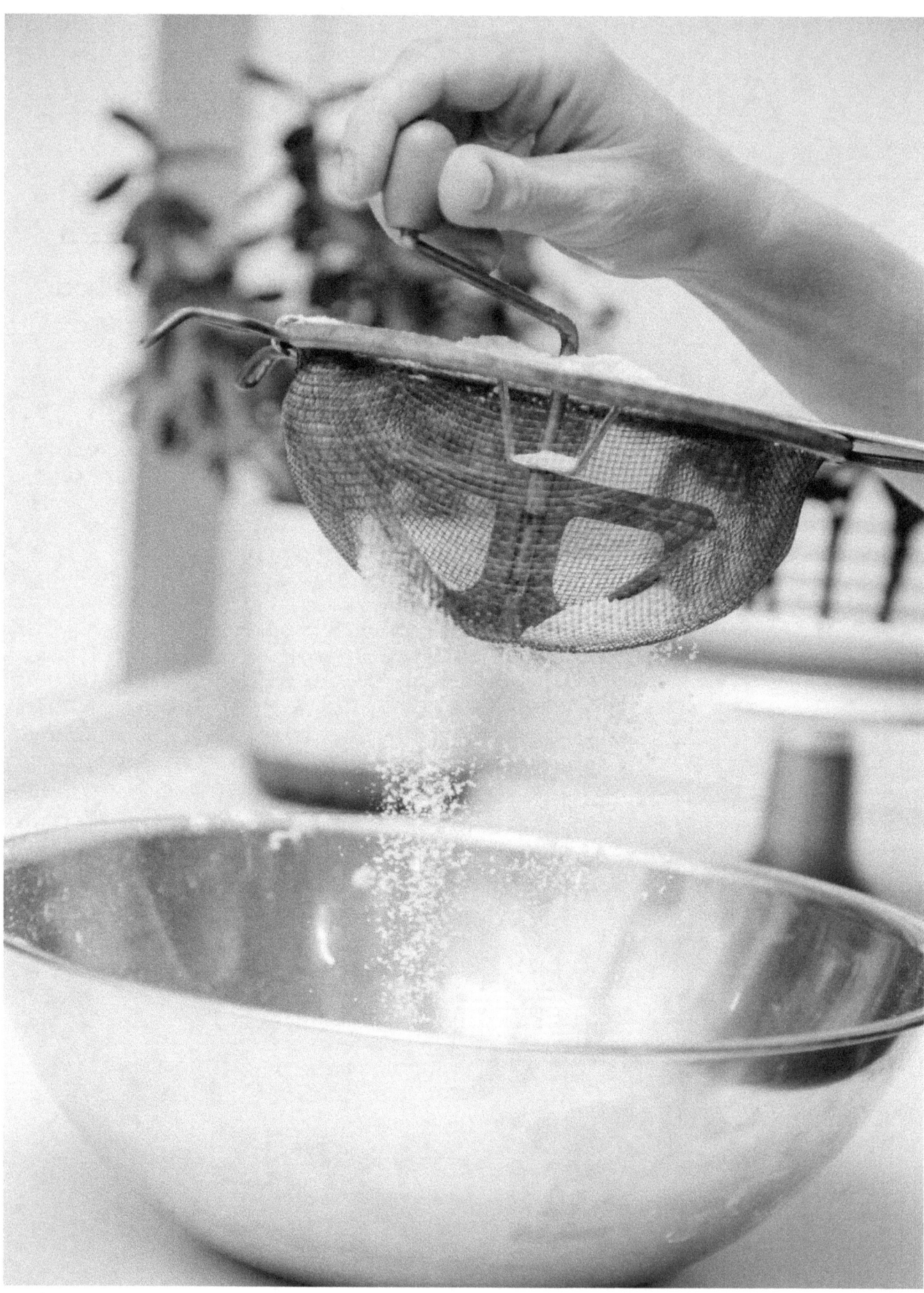

Keto Focaccia Bread

 **Servings:** 8-9

 **Preparation Time:** 55-65 mins

 **Method:** Bake

INGREDIENTS:

- ½ cup coconut flour
- 4 eggs
- 1 teaspoon salt
- 2 teaspoons baking powder
- 1 cup water, boiling
- Herbs of your choice (dried and chopped parsley, oregano, thyme, rosemary etc.), as needed

DIRECTIONS:

1. Preheat an oven to 325°F-162°C. Prepare a baking sheet by lining it with a parchment paper. Grease it with some coconut oil or butter. (You can also use coconut oil cooking spray to grease)
2. Sift the coconut flour, salt, baking powder in a mixing bowl.
3. Stir in the eggs one by one, whisk gently. Add the hot water into it gradually and combine well.
4. Give the dough a focaccia shape. Place the dough over the lined baking sheet, make slits using a knife, top with the herbs, and bake for 30 minutes or until turns golden brown.
5. Take out the baking sheet and allow it to cool down on a wired rack for at least 10-20 minutes.
6. Serve and enjoy!

NUTRITIONAL VALUES (PER SERVING):

Calories: 286
F:18g C:4g fi:1g P:11g

Keto Bacon Bread

Servings:
14-16

Preparation Time:
90-95 mins

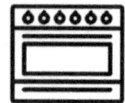

Method:
Bake

INGREDIENTS:

2 teaspoons baking powder

½ teaspoon salt

12 bacon slices (diced)

1 cup coconut flour

2 eggs (lightly beaten)

½ cup unsweetened almond milk

1 Tablespoon butter (melted)

1 teaspoon liquid Stevia

½ cup natural peanut butter, unsweetened

½ cup dry roasted peanuts (chopped)

DIRECTIONS:

1. In a skillet or saucepan of medium size, add the bacon and stir-fry for 7-8 minutes until turns crisp and golden. Drain over paper towel and crumble into small pieces.
2. Preheat an oven to 350°F-176°C. Prepare a medium-size bread pan or loaf pan by greasing it with some coconut oil or butter. (You can also use coconut oil cooking spray to grease)
3. In a mixing bowl, mix the coconut flour, baking powder, and salt until thoroughly combine.
4. In another bowl, beat the eggs, sweetener, milk and butter. Add the peanut butter and beat again.
5. Combine both mixtures with each other. Add the bacon and peanuts; combine well until smooth batter is formed without any visible lumps.
6. Take the prepared batter and slowly pour it in the greased bread or loaf pan; mounding batter slightly in the center so that it creates a rounded top.
7. Place the bread or loaf pan in the preheated oven and bake for 55-60 minutes or until turns golden brown. You can check by inserting a toothpick; when the bread is baked well, toothpick comes out clean.
8. Take out the bread pan and allow it to cool down on a wired rack for at least 10-20 minutes. Shake the pan gently and take out

NUTRITIONAL VALUES (PER SERVING):

Calories:218
F:16g C:10g fi:4g P:9g

Macadamia Magic Bread

Servings:
6-8

Preparation Time:
70-80 mins

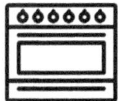

Method:
Bake

INGREDIENTS:

1 cup macadamia seeds

2 egg whites

¼ cup almond flour

v cup ghee

2 Tablespoons flax seeds, ground

1 Tablespoon apple cider vinegar

1 teaspoon baking soda

¾ teaspoon Himalayan salt

4 eggs

DIRECTIONS:

1. Preheat an oven to 350°F-176°C. Prepare a medium-size bread pan or loaf pan by greasing it with some coconut oil or butter. (You can also use coconut oil cooking spray to grease)
2. Add the macadamia seeds in a blender or food processor and process until it has a flour consistency.
3. Add the flax seeds, salt, almond flour, baking soda; blend until well-combined.
4. Whisk the egg whites, apple cider vinegar, egg and ghee in a mixing bowl.
5. Combine both mixtures with each other. Combine well until smooth batter is formed without any visible lumps.
6. Take the prepared batter and slowly pour it in the greased bread or loaf pan; mounding batter slightly in the center so that it creates a rounded top.
7. Place the bread or loaf pan in the preheated oven and bake for 45-50 minutes or until turns golden brown. You can check by inserting a toothpick; when the bread is baked well, toothpick comes out clean.
8. Take out the bread pan and allow it to cool down on a wired rack for at least 10-20 minutes. Shake the pan gently and take out the bread from the pan.
9. Cut into slices and serve!

NUTRITIONAL VALUES (PER SERVING):

Calories:231
F:21g C:2g Fi:0g P:12g

Wholesome Broccoli Bread

Servings:
10

Preparation Time:
40 mins

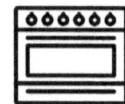

Method:
Bake

INGREDIENTS:

¾ cup broccoli florets, finely chopped

4 Tablespoons coconut flour

1 teaspoon salt

1 cup cheddar cheese, shredded

5 eggs, whisked

2 teaspoons baking powder

DIRECTIONS:

1. Preheat an oven to 350°F-176°C. Prepare a medium-size bread pan or loaf pan by greasing it with some coconut oil or butter. (You can also use coconut oil cooking spray to grease)
2. In a mixing bowl, whisk the egg. In another bowl, add the broccoli, flour and other ingredients; combine well.
3. Combine both mixtures with each other. Combine well until smooth batter is formed without any visible lumps.
4. Take the prepared batter and slowly pour it in the greased bread or loaf pan; mounding batter slightly in the center so that it creates a rounded top.
5. Place the bread or loaf pan in the preheated oven and bake for 15 minutes or until turns golden brown. You can check by inserting a toothpick; when the bread is baked well, toothpick comes out clean.
6. Take out the bread pan and allow it to cool down on a wired rack for at least 10-20 minutes. Shake the pan gently and take out the bread from the pan.
7. Cut into slices and serve!

NUTRITIONAL VALUES (PER SERVING):

Calories:103
F:6g C:3g Fi:1g P:6g

Turmeric Baguette Bread

Servings:
8-9

Preparation Time:
55-60 mins

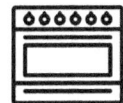
Method:
Bake

INGREDIENTS:

1 cup blanched almond flour

¾ cup psyllium husk powder

1 ½ teaspoons baking soda

2 teaspoon salt

1 teaspoon turmeric

1 cup sifted coconut flour

2 teaspoons xanthan gum

9 egg whites

3 large eggs

¾ cup unsweetened coconut milk

1 cup lukewarm water

½ cup raw cider vinegar

To sprinkle:

¼ teaspoon turmeric

3 Tablespoons blanched almond flour

DIRECTIONS:

1. Preheat an oven to 350°F-176°C. Prepare a baking sheet by lining it with a parchment paper. Grease it with some coconut oil or butter. (You can also use coconut oil cooking spray to grease)
2. In a mixing bowl, combine the almond flour, psyllium husk, turmeric powder, coconut flour, baking soda, salt, and xanthan gum.
3. In another bowl, beat the egg whites, eggs, coconut milk, water, and vinegar.
4. Combine both mixtures with each other. Combine well until smooth batter is formed without any visible lumps. Shape the mixture into two logs/rolls.
5. Combine the turmeric and almond flour in a bowl. Top the rolls with it; make few cuts on top with a knife.
6. Place the logs over the lined baking sheet, give it a loaf shape and bake for 30-40 minutes or until turns golden brown.
7. Take out the baking sheet and allow it to cool down on a wired rack for at least 10-20 minutes.
8. Serve and enjoy!

NUTRITIONAL VALUES (PER SERVING):

Calories:118
F:8g C:5g Fi:1g P:7g

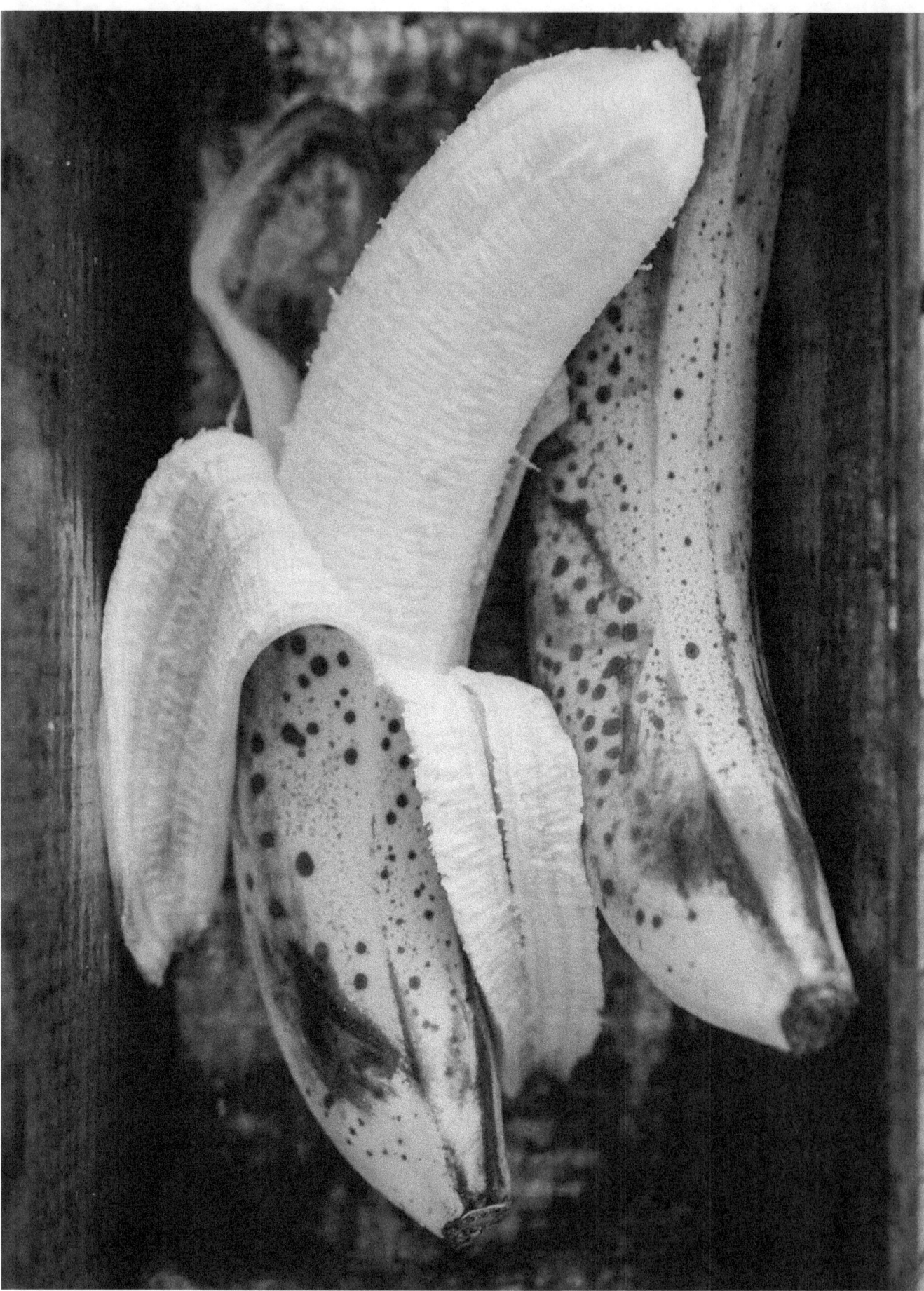

Almond Banana Bread

Servings:
6-8

Preparation Time:
50-60 mins

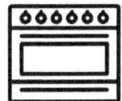

Method:
Bake

INGREDIENTS:

- 7 eggs
- 2 cups almond flour
- ½ cup butter
- 2 Tablespoons olive oil
- 1 teaspoon baking powder
- ½ teaspoon xanthan gum
- ½ teaspoon salt
- 4 drops banana extract
- ¼ cup erythritol
- ¼ cup sunflower seeds
- 2 Tablespoons chia seeds
- 2 Tablespoons sesame seeds (topping)

DIRECTIONS:

1. Preheat an oven to 350°F-176°C. Prepare a medium-size bread pan or loaf pan by greasing it with some coconut oil or butter. (You can also use coconut oil cooking spray to grease)
2. Beat the eggs in a mixing bowl. Add the olive oil and melted butter, continue beating.
3. Add remaining ingredients except for sesame seeds in another mixing bowl. Combine well.
4. Combine both mixtures with each other. Combine well until smooth batter is formed without any visible lumps.
5. Take the prepared batter and slowly pour it in the greased bread or loaf pan; mounding batter slightly in the center so that it creates a rounded top. Add the sesame seeds on top.
6. Place the bread or loaf pan in the preheated oven and bake for 45 minutes or until turns golden brown. You can check by inserting a toothpick; when the bread is baked well, toothpick comes out clean.
7. Take out the bread pan and allow it to cool down on a wired rack for at least 10-20 minutes. Shake the pan gently and take out the bread from the pan.
8. Cut into slices and serve!

NUTRITIONAL VALUES (PER SERVING):

Calories: 276
F:28g C:4g fi:0.5g P:3g

No-Flour Keto Egg Bread

Servings:
4

Preparation Time:
35-40 mins

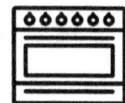

Method:
Bake

INGREDIENTS:

12 ounces almond butter
5 eggs
1 ½ Tablespoon lemon juice
¾ teaspoon baking soda
¼ teaspoon salt

DIRECTIONS:

1. Preheat an oven to 350°F-176°C. Prepare a medium-size bread pan or loaf pan by greasing it with some coconut oil or butter. (You can also use coconut oil cooking spray to grease)
2. Blend the almond butter and eggs until smooth in a mixing bowl. Add the lemon juice and salt; mix well.
3. Add the baking soda and mix again.
4. Take the prepared batter and slowly pour it in the greased bread or loaf pan; mounding batter slightly in the center so that it creates a rounded top.
5. Place the bread or loaf pan in the preheated oven and bake for 30 minutes or until turns golden brown. You can check by inserting a toothpick; when the bread is baked well, toothpick comes out clean.
6. Take out the bread pan and allow it to cool down on a wired rack for at least 10-20 minutes. Shake the pan gently and take out the bread from the pan.
7. Cut into slices and serve!

NUTRITIONAL VALUES (PER SERVING):

Calories:176
F:16g C:5g fi:1g P:9g

Cauliflower Seeded Bread

Servings:
7-8

Preparation Time:
50-60 mins

Method:
Bake

INGREDIENTS:

- 1 cup cauliflower rice
- 5 eggs
- ½ teaspoon sea salt
- ½ teaspoon baking soda
- 2 cups almond flour
- 4 Tablespoons psyllium husk powder

For decoration:

- 1 teaspoon pumpkin seeds
- 1 teaspoon sesame seeds
- 1 teaspoon sunflower seeds

DIRECTIONS:

1. To make the cauliflower rice, chop the cauliflower into large pieces.
2. Grate into cauliflower into rice-like consistency. Sauté for 5-6 minutes over medium cooking flame in a saucepan with 1 Tablespoon olive oil.
3. Preheat an oven to 350°F-176°C. Prepare a medium-size bread pan or loaf pan by greasing it with some coconut oil or butter. (You can also use coconut oil cooking spray to grease)
4. Mix the dry ingredients in a mixing bowl. Beat the eggs and add it with the dry mixture.
5. Add the cauliflower rice. Combine well until smooth batter is formed without any visible lumps.
6. Take the prepared batter and slowly pour it in the greased bread or loaf pan; mounding batter slightly in the center so that it creates a rounded top. Top with the seeds.
7. Place the bread or loaf pan in the preheated oven and bake for 50-55 minutes or until turns golden brown. You can check by inserting a toothpick; when the bread is baked well, toothpick comes out clean.
8. Take out the bread pan and allow it to cool down on a wired rack for at least 10-20 minutes. Shake the pan gently and take out the bread from the pan.
9. Cut into slices and serve!

NUTRITIONAL VALUES (PER SERVING):

Calories:227
F:17g C:6g fi:2g P:7g

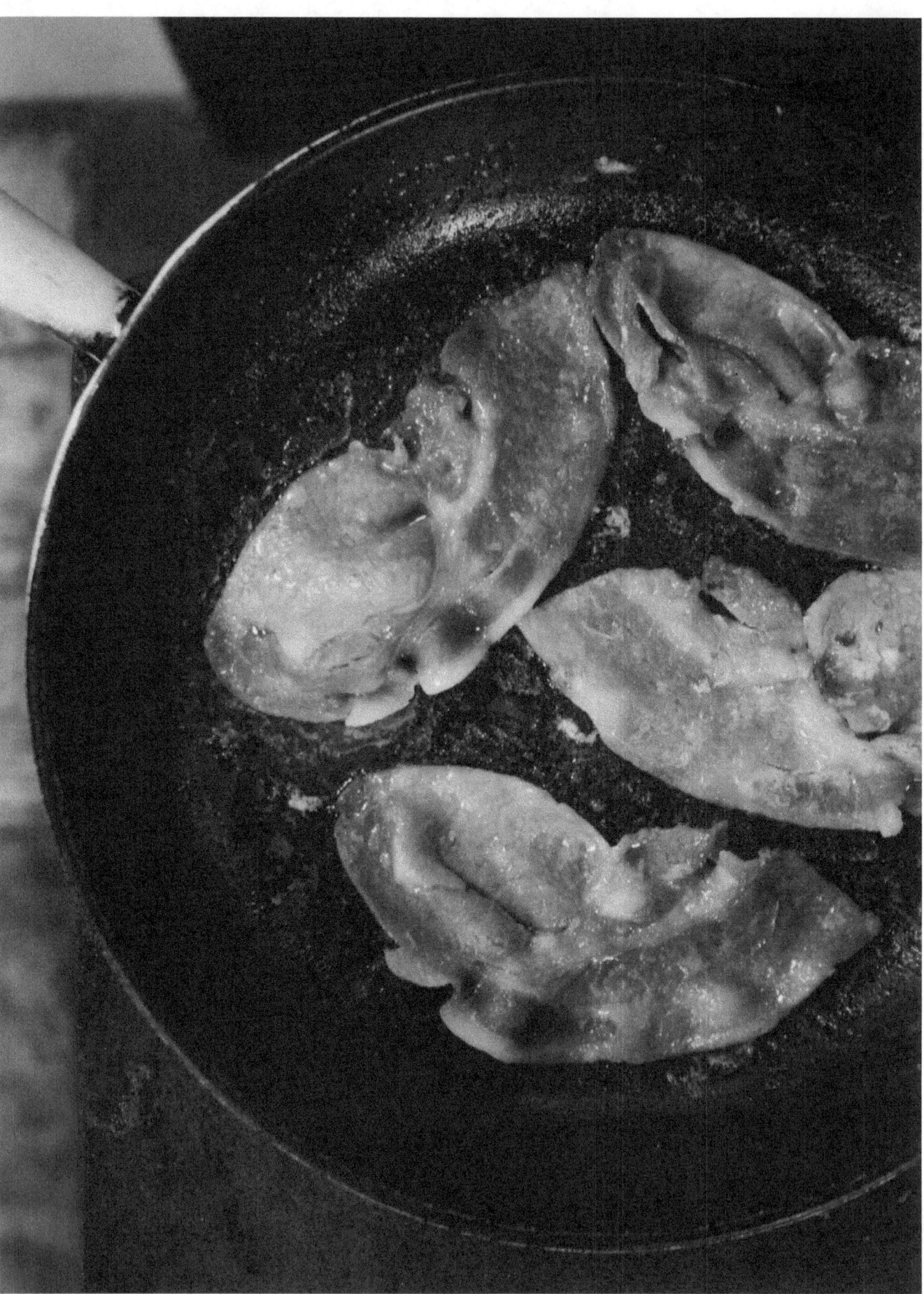

Cheese & Bacon Bread

Servings:
8-10

Preparation Time:
60-70 mins

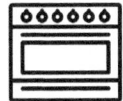
Method:
Bake

INGREDIENTS:

1 cup cheddar cheese, grated finely

⅓ cup sour cream

1 ½ almond flour

2 eggs

7 ½ ounce bacon strips

4 Tablespoons butter

1 Tablespoon baking powder

DIRECTIONS:

1. Preheat an oven to 300°F-148°C. Prepare a medium-size bread pan or loaf pan by greasing it with some coconut oil or butter. (You can also use coconut oil cooking spray to grease)
2. In a skillet or saucepan of medium size, add the bacon and some olive oil, and stir-fry until turns crisp and golden. Drain over paper towel and crumble into small pieces.
3. Combine the almond flour and baking powder in a mixing bowl. Whisk the sour cream and eggs in another bowl.
4. Combine both mixtures with each other.
5. Add the cooked bacon, cheese, and melted butter. Combine well until smooth batter is formed without any visible lumps.
6. Take the prepared batter and slowly pour it in the greased bread or loaf pan; mounding batter slightly in the center so that it creates a rounded top.
7. Place the bread or loaf pan in the preheated oven and bake for 45-50 minutes or until turns golden brown. You can check by inserting a toothpick; when the bread is baked well, toothpick comes out clean.
8. Take out the bread pan and allow it to cool down on a wired rack for at least 10-20 minutes. Shake the pan gently and take out the bread from the pan.
9. Cut into slices and serve!

NUTRITIONAL VALUES (PER SERVING):

Calories:193
F:26g C:3g fi:0.5g P:10g

Zucchini Zeal Bread

Servings:
4

Preparation Time:
80-90 mins

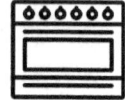

Method:
Bake

INGREDIENTS:

1 teaspoon baking powder

¼ teaspoon cinnamon

1 medium zucchini (peeled and finely shredded)

½ cup almond flour

¼ cup coconut flour

¼ teaspoon salt

4 eggs (lightly beaten)

½ cup coconut oil

1 teaspoon vanilla extract

1 teaspoon lemon zest

DIRECTIONS:

1. Preheat an oven to 350°F-176°C. Prepare a medium-size bread pan or loaf pan by greasing it with some coconut oil or butter. (You can also use coconut oil cooking spray to grease)
2. In a mixing bowl, whisk the almond flour, coconut flour, baking powder, cinnamon, and salt until thoroughly combined.
3. In another mixing bowl, whisk the eggs, coconut oil, vanilla extract, and lemon zest. Add the zucchini and mix again.
4. Combine both mixtures with each other. Combine well until smooth batter is formed without any visible lumps.
5. Take the prepared batter and slowly pour it in the greased bread or loaf pan; mounding batter slightly in the center so that it creates a rounded top.
6. Place the bread or loaf pan in the preheated oven and bake for 50 minutes or until turns golden brown. You can check by inserting a toothpick; when the bread is baked well, toothpick comes out clean.
7. Take out the bread pan and allow it to cool down on a wired rack for at least 10-20 minutes. Shake the pan gently and take out the bread from the pan.
8. Cut into slices and serve!

NUTRITIONAL VALUES (PER SERVING):

Calories:223
F:20g C:5g fi:0.5g P:5g

Cashew Butter Bread

Servings:
8-10

Preparation Time:
60-70 mins

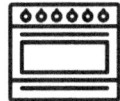

Method:
Bake

INGREDIENTS:

1 cup cashew butter

2 teaspoons apple cider vinegar

2 teaspoons baking soda

5 eggs (lightly beaten)

¼ teaspoon salt

DIRECTIONS:

1. Preheat an oven to 350°F-176°C. Prepare a medium-size bread pan or loaf pan by greasing it with some coconut oil or butter. (You can also use coconut oil cooking spray to grease)
2. Beat the cashew butter and eggs in a mixing bowl until turn smooth. Add the apple cider vinegar and beat more.
3. Add baking soda and salt; mix to make a smooth batter.
4. Take the prepared batter and slowly pour it in the greased bread or loaf pan; mounding batter slightly in the center so that it creates a rounded top.
5. Place the bread or loaf pan in the preheated oven and bake for 40-50 minutes or until turns golden brown. You can check by inserting a toothpick; when the bread is baked well, toothpick comes out clean.
6. Take out the bread pan and allow it to cool down on a wired rack for at least 10-20 minutes. Shake the pan gently and take out the bread from the pan.
7. Cut into slices and serve!

NUTRITIONAL VALUES (PER SERVING):

Calories:176
F:14g C:6g Fi:0g P:8g

Jalapeno Delight Bread

Servings:
70-80

Preparation Time:
4-6 mins

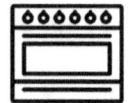

Method:
Bake

INGREDIENTS:

3 jalapenos, sliced
¼ teaspoon baking soda
6 eggs, large
4 ounce bacon strips
¼ cup water
½ cup ghee
½ teaspoon salt
½ cup coconut flour sifted

DIRECTIONS:

1. Preheat an oven to 400°F-204°C. Prepare a medium-size bread pan or loaf pan by greasing it with some coconut oil or butter. (You can also use coconut oil cooking spray to grease)
2. Add the jalapenos and bacon in another greased small baking pan; roast for 8-10 minutes, flipping it between. Take out and remove the seeds.
3. Add the bacon and jalapeno in a food processor and pulse until they are finely crumbled.
4. Combine the ghee, egg, coconut flour and water in a mixing bowl. Add the jalapeno mixture into the batter.
5. Combine well until smooth batter is formed without any visible lumps.
6. Take the prepared batter and slowly pour it in the greased bread or loaf pan; mounding batter slightly in the center so that it creates a rounded top.
7. Place the bread or loaf pan in the preheated oven and bake for 45 minutes or until turns golden brown. You can check by inserting a toothpick; when the bread is baked well, toothpick comes out clean.
8. Take out the bread pan and allow it to cool down on a wired rack for at least 10-20 minutes. Shake the pan gently and take out the bread from the pan.
9. Cut into slices and serve!

NUTRITIONAL VALUES (PER SERVING):

Calories:328
F:28g C:3g fi:0g P:13g

Cream Onion Bread

Servings:
12-14

Preparation Time:
70-80 mins

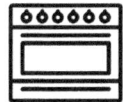

Method:
Bake

INGREDIENTS:

- 1 cup sharp cheddar, grated
- 2 ½ teaspoon baking powder
- ¼ cup heavy whipping cream
- ½ teaspoon baking soda
- ¼ cup olive oil
- 1 teaspoon xanthan gum
- ¼ cup butter
- 4 eggs
- 12 ounces cream cheese
- ½ onion, sliced and caramelized
- 1-2 teaspoon liquid stevia
- ¼ teaspoon cream of tartar

DIRECTIONS:

1. Preheat an oven to 350°F-176°C. Prepare a medium-size bread pan or loaf pan by lining it with a parchment paper. Grease it with some coconut oil or butter. (You can also use coconut oil cooking spray to grease)
2. Caramelize the onions with some coconut oil in a saucepan and set aside.
3. Combine the cream cheese and butter in a heat-proof bowl and microwave it for 45-50 seconds.
4. Add the whipping cream, olive oil, and liquid stevia in a mixing bowl and mix well.
5. Whisk the eggs and cream of tartar in another mixing bowl until turn frothy. Add the cheese mixture and whisk it again.
6. Add the cheddar cheese and the onions; combine well. In another bowl, combine the baking powder, salt, xanthan gum, and baking soda.
7. Combine the mixtures and combine well until smooth batter is formed without any visible lumps.
8. Take the prepared batter and slowly pour it in the greased bread or loaf pan; mounding batter slightly in the center so that it creates a rounded top.
9. Place the bread or loaf pan in the preheated oven and bake for 50-55 minutes or until turns golden brown. You can check by inserting a toothpick; when the bread is baked well, toothpick comes out clean.
10. Take out the bread pan and allow it to cool down on a wired rack for at least 10-20 minutes. Shake the pan gently and take out the bread from the pan.
11. Cut into slices and serve!

NUTRITIONAL VALUES (PER SERVING):

Calories:157
F:11g C:2g fi:0g P:12g

Amazing Fougasse Bread

Servings:
5-6

Preparation Time:
40-45 mins

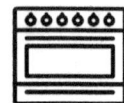

Method:
Bake

INGREDIENTS:

1 large egg

10 olives, chopped

2 Tablespoons olive oil

2 Tablespoons salt

1 Tablespoon dried basil

1 Tablespoon coconut flour, sifted

1 cup blanched almond flour

2 teaspoons ground chia seeds

1 ½ Tablespoons water

1 cup grated mozzarella cheese

3 Tablespoons cream cheese

DIRECTIONS:

1. Preheat an oven to 350ºF-176ºC. Prepare a baking sheet by lining it with a parchment paper. Grease it with some coconut oil or butter. (You can also use coconut oil cooking spray to grease)
2. Combine the chia seeds and water in a bowl. Place aside for 15 minutes.
3. Combine the cream cheese and mozzarella cheese in a heatproof bowl. Melt in a microwave.
4. In another bowl, ass the almond flour, egg, chia seeds mixture, chopped olives, basil, and salt; combine well. Add the melted cheese and combine again.
5. Place the mixture over the lined baking sheet, spread it into a leaf like shape. Take a knife and make a 2-3 cuts across the leaf shapes (cut the whole dough completely). Using finger, open the cuts, and top the bread with some coconut flour and salt.
6. Bake for 10 minutes or until turns golden brown.
7. Take out the baking sheet and allow it to cool down on a wired rack for at least 10-20 minutes.
8. Brush with some olive oil. Serve and enjoy!

NUTRITIONAL VALUES (PER SERVING):

Calories: 227
F: 20g C: 4g fi: 0g P: 9g

Keto Corn Bread

Servings:
4

Preparation Time:
35-40 mins

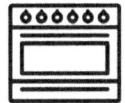

Method:
Bake

INGREDIENTS:

- ¼ cup yellow cornmeal
- ¾ cup almond flour
- ¼ cup coconut flour
- 1 teaspoon salt
- 3 eggs (lightly beaten)
- ½ cup coconut milk
- 2 teaspoons baking powder
- 3 Tablespoons vegetable oil coconut flour

DIRECTIONS:

1. Preheat an oven to 350°F-176°C. Prepare a medium-size bread pan or loaf pan by greasing it with some coconut oil or butter. (You can also use coconut oil cooking spray to grease)
2. In a mixing bowl, combine the almond flour, coconut flour, cornmeal, baking powder, and salt until thoroughly combined.
3. In another mixing bowl, whisk the eggs, coconut milk, and vegetable oil until thoroughly combined.
4. Combine both mixtures with each other. Combine well until smooth batter is formed without any visible lumps.
5. Take the prepared batter and slowly pour it in the greased bread or loaf pan; mounding batter slightly in the center so that it creates a rounded top.
6. Place the bread or loaf pan in the preheated oven and bake for 20 minutes or until turns golden brown. You can check by inserting a toothpick; when the bread is baked well, toothpick comes out clean.
7. Take out the bread pan and allow it to cool down on a wired rack for at least 10-20 minutes. Shake the pan gently and take out the bread from the pan.
8. Cut into slices and serve!

NUTRITIONAL VALUES (PER SERVING):

Calories:159
F:12g C:8g Fi:3g P:5g

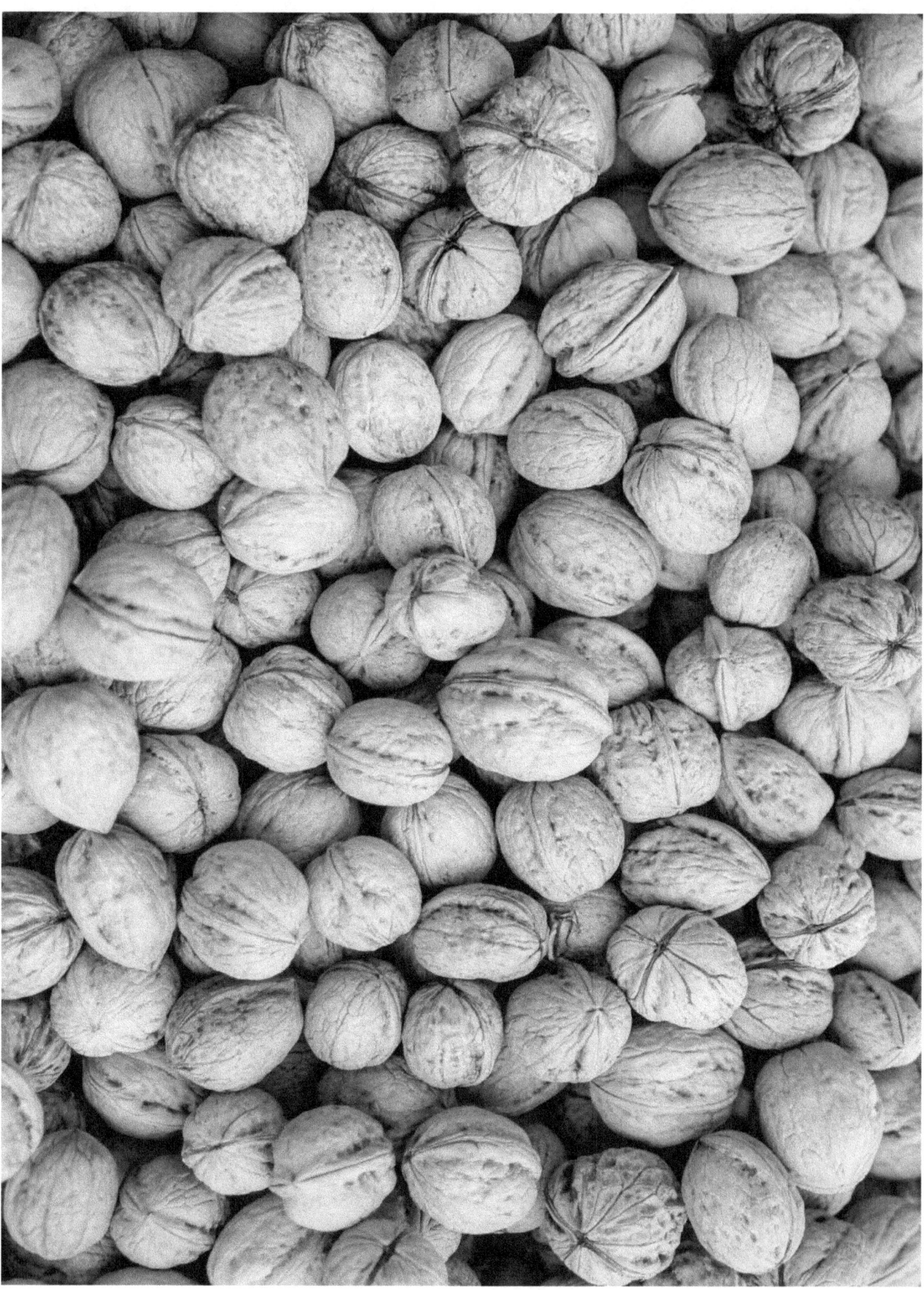

Walnut Zucchini Bread

Servings:
6-8

Preparation Time:
80-70 mins

Method:
Bake

INGREDIENTS:

1 teaspoon psyllium husk powder

8 Tablespoons coconut flour

8 walnuts, coarsely chopped

½ teaspoon salt

8 Tablespoons butter

6 eggs

1 medium zucchini, peeled and finely grated

DIRECTIONS:

1. Preheat an oven to 350°F-176°C. Prepare a medium-size bread pan or loaf pan by greasing it with some coconut oil or butter. (You can also use coconut oil cooking spray to grease)
2. Mix the coconut flour, psyllium husk powder, butter, salt and zucchini in a mixing bowl.
3. Beat the eggs and mix with the flour mixture.
4. Combine both mixtures with each other. Combine well until smooth batter is formed without any visible lumps.
5. Take the prepared batter and slowly pour it in the greased bread or loaf pan; mounding batter slightly in the center so that it creates a rounded top. Add the walnuts on top.
6. Place the bread or loaf pan in the preheated oven and bake for 50 minutes or until turns golden brown. You can check by inserting a toothpick; when the bread is baked well, toothpick comes out clean.
7. Take out the bread pan and allow it to cool down on a wired rack for at least 10-20 minutes. Shake the pan gently and take out the bread from the pan.
8. Cut into slices and serve!

NUTRITIONAL VALUES (PER SERVING):

Calories:187
F:16g C:5g Fi:2g P:6g

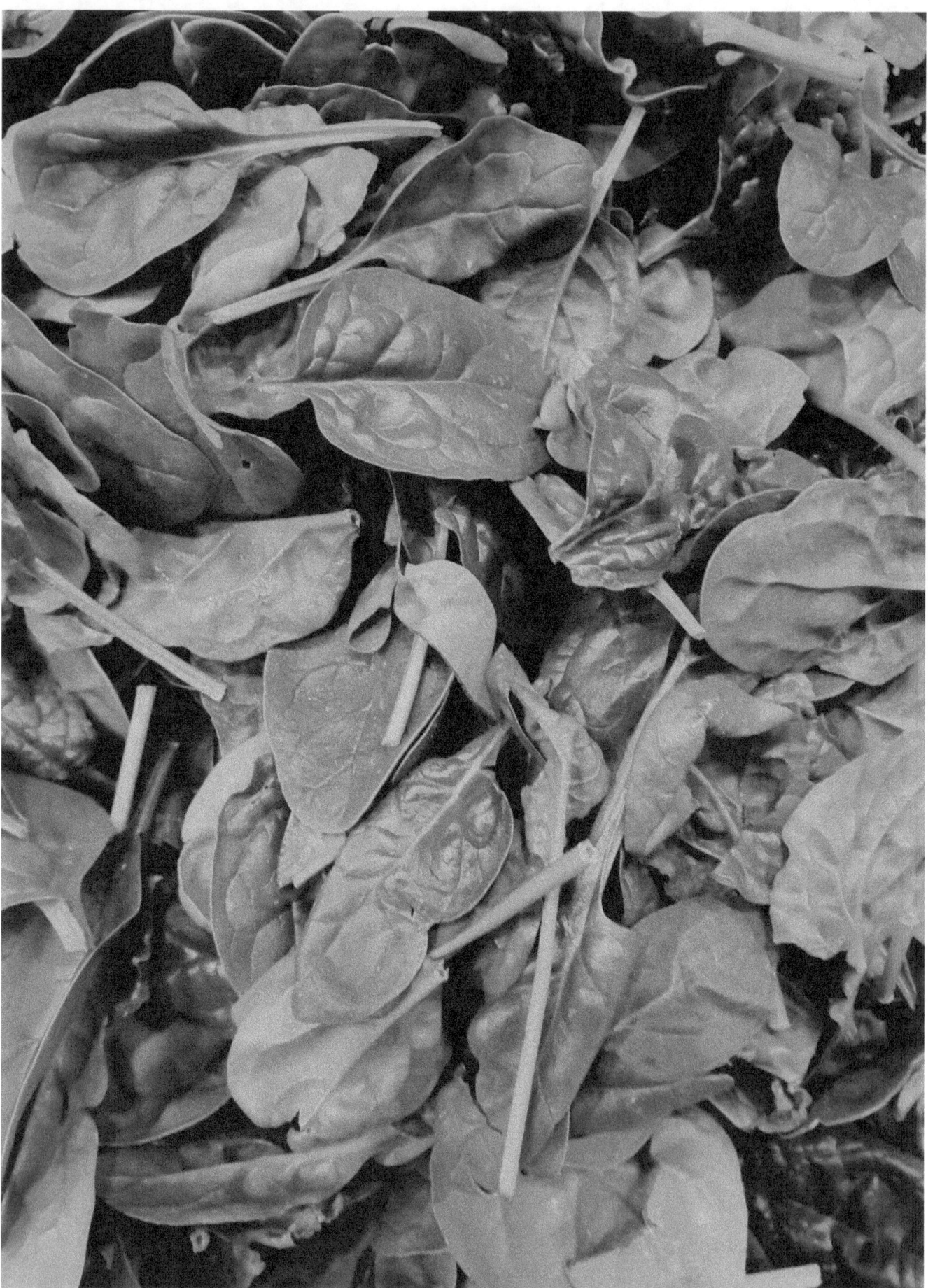

Spinach Cheese Bread

Servings:
4-5

Preparation Time:
25-30 mins

Method:
Bake

INGREDIENTS:

10 ounce chopped spinach leaves

4 eggs, beaten

1/4 teaspoon garlic powder

1/4 teaspoon salt

1/8 teaspoon pepper

1 ounce parmesan cheese, shredded

DIRECTIONS:

9. Preheat an oven to 400ºF-204ºC. Prepare a medium-size bread pan or loaf pan by greasing it with some coconut oil or butter. (You can also use coconut oil cooking spray to grease)
10. Beat the eggs in a bowl. In another bowl, combine remaining ingredients.
11. Combine both mixtures with each other. Combine well until smooth batter is formed without any visible lumps.
12. Take the prepared batter and slowly pour it in the greased bread or loaf pan; mounding batter slightly in the center so that it creates a rounded top.
13. Place the bread or loaf pan in the preheated oven and bake for 15-20 minutes or until turns golden brown. You can check by inserting a toothpick; when the bread is baked well, toothpick comes out clean.
14. Take out the bread pan and allow it to cool down on a wired rack for at least 10-20 minutes. Shake the pan gently and take out the bread from the pan.
15. Cut into slices and serve!

NUTRITIONAL VALUES (PER SERVING):

Calories: 81
F:5g C:1g fi:0g P:7g

Round Cream Bread

Servings:
3-4

Preparation Time:
20 mins

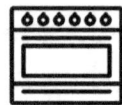

Method:
Bake

INGREDIENTS:

3 eggs, separated

3 Tablespoons cream cheese, room temperature

½ teaspoon baking powder

Salt to taste

DIRECTIONS:

1. Preheat an oven to 300ºF-148ºC. Prepare a baking sheet by lining it with a parchment paper. Grease it with some coconut oil or butter. (You can also use coconut oil cooking spray to grease)
2. In a mixing bowl, combine the egg yolks, cream cheese and salt. In another bowl, whisk the egg whites and baking powder.
3. Combine both mixtures with each other. Combine well until smooth batter is formed without any visible lumps.
4. Place one Tablespoon batter over the lined baking sheet, spread using a spoon into a round, repeat with remaining batter, and bake for 15-20 minutes or until turns golden brown.
5. Take out the baking sheet and allow it to cool down on a wired rack for at least 10-20 minutes.
6. Serve and enjoy!

NUTRITIONAL VALUES (PER SERVING):

Calories:148
F:12g C:1g Fi:0g P:8g

Cream Onion Keto Bread

Servings:
4

Preparation Time:
20 mins

Method:
Bake

INGREDIENTS:

1 Tablespoon apple vinegar

3 Tablespoons spring onions, minced

3 Tablespoons cream cheese

3 eggs, whites and yolk separated

Salt to taste

DIRECTIONS:

1. Preheat an oven to 300°F-148°C. Prepare a baking sheet by lining it with a parchment paper. Grease it with some coconut oil or butter. (You can also use coconut oil cooking spray to grease)
2. In a mixing bowl, combine the egg yolks, cream cheese, minced onions and salt. In another bowl, whisk the egg whites and vinegar.
3. Combine both mixtures with each other. Combine well until smooth batter is formed without any visible lumps.
4. Place one Tablespoon batter over the lined baking sheet, spread using a spoon into a round, repeat with remaining batter, and bake for 15-20 minutes or until turns golden brown.
5. Take out the baking sheet and allow it to cool down on a wired rack for at least 10-20 minutes.
6. Serve and enjoy!

NUTRITIONAL VALUES (PER SERVING):

Calories:148
F:12g C:2g fi:0g P:5g

Mug Mystery Bread

Servings:
1

Preparation Time:
10 mins

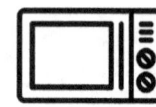

Method:
Microwave

INGREDIENTS:

1/4 cup almond flour
1 teaspoon olive oil
1 teaspoon butter
1 egg (lightly beaten)
½ teaspoon baking powder
Salt to taste

DIRECTIONS:

1. Take a mug and grease inside surface with melted butter.
2. In a mixing bowl, whisk the eggs; add the almond flour, oil, and baking powder. Combine well.
3. Add the batter into a mug.
4. Set microwave to its highest temperature setting. Place the mug and microwave for 2-3 minutes, or until the top portion of golden brown.
5. Cool down completely and using a knife, carve out the bread.

NUTRITIONAL VALUES
(PER SERVING):

Calories:324
F:26g C:6g fi:1g P:12g

CHAPTER 3
KETO MUFFINS

Chocolate Cream Muffins

Servings:
8

Preparation Time:
30-45 mins

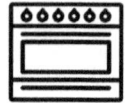

Method:
Bake

INGREDIENTS:

2 cups blanched almond flour

2 teaspoons baking powder

10 drops liquid stevia

1 pinch salt

½ cup melted butter or coconut oil

¼ cup powdered erythritol

1 teaspoon vanilla extract

4 large eggs

¼ cup water

Drizzle:

2 Tablespoons cocoa powder

4 Tablespoons cocoa butter, melted

3 Tablespoons heavy cream

2 Tablespoons cream cheese

5 drops liquid stevia

DIRECTIONS:

1. Preheat an oven to 350°F-176°C. Take 8 muffins pans or a muffin tray; grease one by one with some coconut oil or butter. (You can also use coconut oil cooking spray to grease)
2. In a large bowl, combine the almond flour, baking powder, erythritol, and salt.
3. In another bowl, beat the eggs; add the melted butter, vanilla, and stevia drops, and mix well.
4. Combine both mixtures with each other. Combine well until smooth batter is formed without any visible lumps.
5. Add the prepared batter evenly in the greased muffin pans or a tray; bake for 15-20 minutes or until turns golden brown. You can check by inserting a toothpick; when the bread is baked well, toothpick comes out clean.
6. In a mixing bowl, combine heavy cream, cream cheese, and stevia.
7. In another bowl, add the cocoa powder and butter. Combine well.
8. Take out and allow to cool down on a wired rack for at least 10-20 minutes. Add the cocoa mix on top on the muffins and then add the cream mixture. Serve and enjoy.

NUTRITIONAL VALUES (PER SERVING):

Calories: 289
F:16g C:5g fi:2g P:8g

Bacon Bake Muffins

Servings:
12

Preparation Time:
25-30 mins

Method:
Bake

INGREDIENTS:

- 4 eggs
- ½ cup ghee (melted)
- 3 cups almond flour
- 1 cup bacon bits
- 2 teaspoons lemon thyme
- 1 teaspoon baking soda

DIRECTIONS:

1. Preheat an oven to 350°F-176°C. Take 12 muffins pans or a muffin tray; grease one by one with some coconut oil or butter. (You can also use coconut oil cooking spray to grease)
2. Combine the ghee, almond flour, baking soda, eggs and lemon thyme in a mixing bowl. Add the bacon bits and combine well.
3. Add the prepared batter evenly in the greased muffin pans or a tray; bake for 20 minutes or until turns golden brown. You can check by inserting a toothpick; when the bread is baked well, toothpick comes out clean.
4. Take out and allow to cool down on a wired rack for at least 10-20 minutes. Serve and enjoy.

NUTRITIONAL VALUES (PER SERVING):

Calories: 194
F:23g C:4g Fi:1g P:10g

Choco Pecan Muffins

Servings:
8

Preparation Time:
40-45 mins

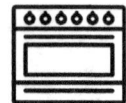

Method:
Bake

INGREDIENTS:

1 cup pecan, chopped coarsely

½ cup butter

2 ½ ounce cacao chocolate, chopped

1 cup almond flour

1 teaspoon liquid Stevia

2 eggs

Pinch of salt

DIRECTIONS:

1. Preheat an oven to 325°F-162°C. Take 8 muffins pans or a muffin tray; grease one by one with some coconut oil or butter. (You can also use coconut oil cooking spray to grease)
2. Combine the sweetener, pecans, almond flour and salt in a mixing bowl.
3. In another mixing bowl, whisk the eggs and butter until turns fluffy.
4. Combine both mixtures with each other. Combine well until smooth batter is formed without any visible lumps. Mix in the chocolate.
5. Add the prepared batter evenly in the greased muffin pans or a tray; bake for 25-30 minutes or until turns golden brown. You can check by inserting a toothpick; when the bread is baked well, toothpick comes out clean.
6. Take out and allow to cool down on a wired rack for at least 10-20 minutes. Serve and enjoy.

NUTRITIONAL VALUES (PER SERVING):

Calories:263
F:24g C:4g fi:0.5g P:4g

Cinnamon Pumpkin Muffins

Servings:
6-8

Preparation Time:
20-25 mins

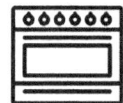

Method:
Bake

INGREDIENTS:

- 1 Tablespoon cinnamon
- ½ cup cashew, almond or coconut butter
- ½ cup almond flour
- ½ cup coconut oil
- 1 teaspoon baking powder
- ½ cup pumpkin puree

Glaze:

- ¼ cup coconut butter
- 2 teaspoons lemon juice
- ¼ cup almond or coconut milk
- 10-15 drops liquid Stevia

DIRECTIONS:

1. Preheat an oven to 350°F-176°C. Take 6-8 muffins pans or a muffin tray; grease one by one with some coconut oil or butter. (You can also use coconut oil cooking spray to grease)
2. In a mixing bowl, combine the dry ingredients. In another bowl, combine the wet ingredients.
3. Combine both mixtures with each other. Combine well until smooth batter is formed without any visible lumps.
4. Add the prepared batter evenly in the greased muffin pans or a tray; bake for 15 minutes or until turns golden brown. You can check by inserting a toothpick; when the bread is baked well, toothpick comes out clean.
5. Take out and allow to cool down on a wired rack for at least 10-20 minutes. In a bowl, combine all glaze ingredients and mix well until smooth.
6. Top the muffins with prepared glaze. Serve and enjoy.

NUTRITIONAL VALUES (PER SERVING):

Calories:107
F:9g C:3g fi:0g P:5g

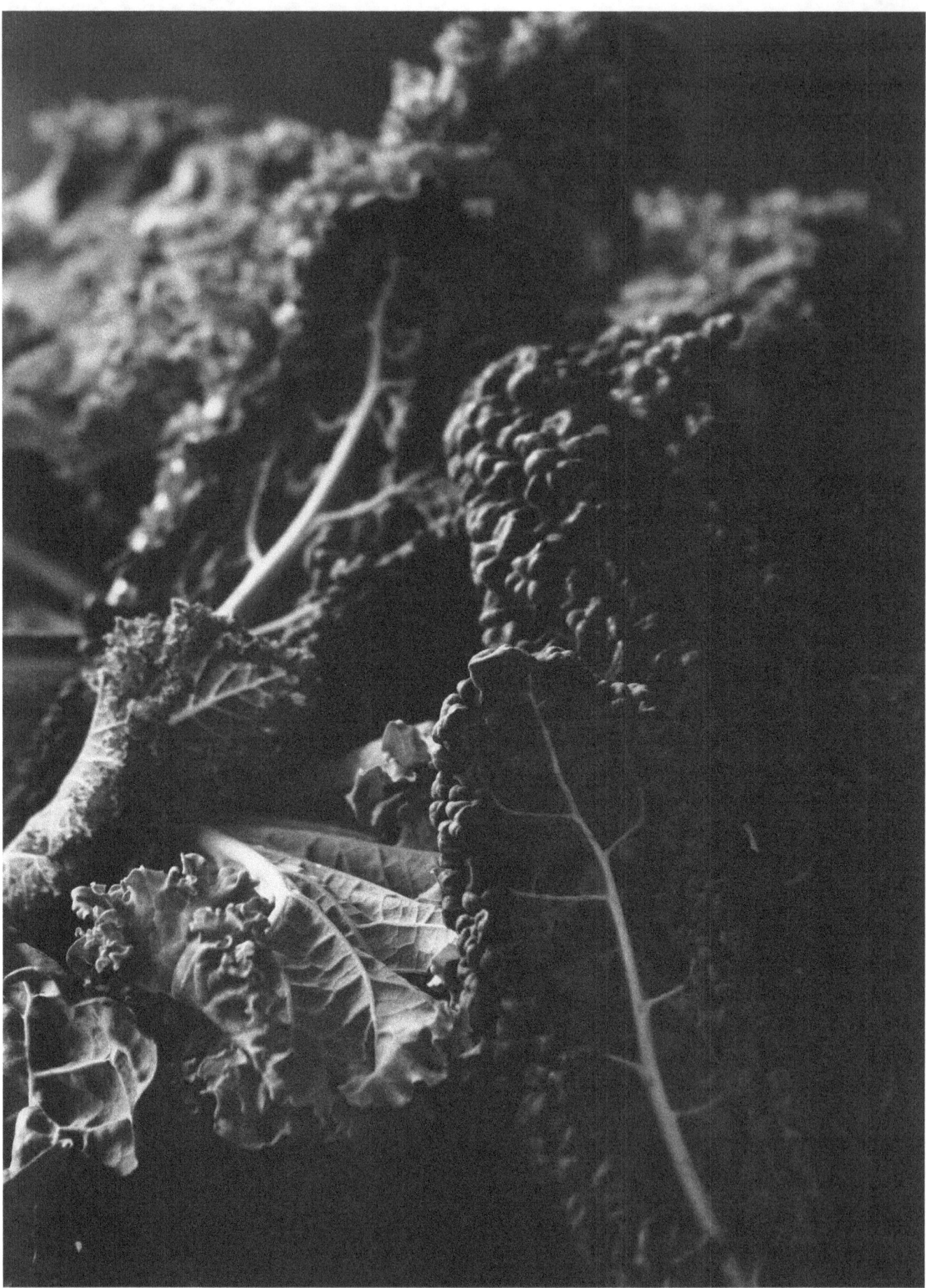

Almond Kale Muffins

Servings:
8

Preparation Time:
40-45 mins

Method:
Bake

INGREDIENTS:

6 eggs
½ cup almond milk
1 cup kale (finely chopped)
¼ cup chives (finely chopped)
Salt and black pepper to taste

DIRECTIONS:

1. Preheat an oven to 350°F-176°C. Take 8 muffins pans or a muffin tray; grease one by one with some coconut oil or butter. (You can also use coconut oil cooking spray to grease)
2. Beat the eggs in a mixing bowl. Add the kale and chives; combine well. Add the coconut milk, salt and pepper. Combine well until smooth batter is formed without any visible lumps.
3. Add the prepared batter evenly in the greased muffin pans or a tray; bake for 30 minutes or until turns golden brown. You can check by inserting a toothpick; when the bread is baked well, toothpick comes out clean.
4. Take out and allow to cool down on a wired rack for at least 10-20 minutes. Serve and enjoy.

NUTRITIONAL VALUES
(PER SERVING):

Calories:235
F:19g C:5g Fi:1g P:13g

Pumpkin Cinnamon Muffins

Servings:
6-8

Preparation Time:
40-45 mins

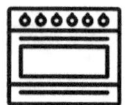

Method:
Bake

INGREDIENTS:

2 cups pumpkin seeds, ground

Dash of cinnamon

4 eggs, separated

¾ cup coconut sugar

1 teaspoon baking powder

DIRECTIONS:

1. Preheat an oven to 350°F-176°C. Take 6-8 muffins pans or a muffin tray; grease one by one with some coconut oil or butter. (You can also use coconut oil cooking spray to grease)
2. Whisk the egg whites in a mixing bowl with ½ cup coconut sugar until becomes foamy. In another bowl, whisk the egg yolks and remaining coconut sugar.
3. Combine all dry ingredients in another mixing bowl. Combine all the mixtures with each other. Combine well until smooth batter is formed without any visible lumps.
4. Add the prepared batter evenly in the greased muffin pans or a tray; bake for 30 minutes or until turns golden brown. You can check by inserting a toothpick; when the bread is baked well, toothpick comes out clean.
5. Take out and allow to cool down on a wired rack for at least 10-20 minutes. Serve and enjoy.

NUTRITIONAL VALUES (PER SERVING):

Calories:286
F:24g C:11g fi:4g P:19g

Keto Veggie Muffins

Servings:
6-8

Preparation Time:
25-30 mins

Method:
Bake

INGREDIENTS:

½ cup green peas, crushed

¼ cup grated carrots

½ cup bell pepper, finely chopped

5 eggs

½ cup full-fat cheese or your choice, grated

Salt and black pepper to taste

DIRECTIONS:

1. Preheat an oven to 375ºF-190ºC. Take 6-8 muffins pans or a muffin tray; grease one by one with some coconut oil or butter. (You can also use coconut oil cooking spray to grease)
2. Combine the vegetables in a mixing bowl and season with salt and black pepper.
3. Whisk the eggs in a mixing bowl. Mix in the vegetable mixture; combine well until smooth batter is formed without any visible lumps.
4. Add the prepared batter evenly in the greased muffin pans or a tray; top with the cheese.
5. Bake for 15-20 minutes or until turns golden brown. You can check by inserting a toothpick; when the bread is baked well, toothpick comes out clean.
6. Take out and allow to cool down on a wired rack for at least 10-20 minutes. Serve and enjoy.

NUTRITIONAL VALUES (PER SERVING):

Calories:92
F:8g C:3g Fi:1g P:7g

Sausage Oregano Muffins

Servings:
12

Preparation Time:
35-40 mins

Method:
Bake

INGREDIENTS:

¾ cup red bell pepper (finely chopped)

8 ounces pork sausage

9 eggs

1 ½ cups chopped spinach

¼ cup coconut milk

½ sweet onion (thinly sliced)

1 Tablespoon extra-virgin olive oil

1 teaspoon fresh oregano (chopped)

¾ teaspoon salt

Ground pepper to taste

DIRECTIONS:

1. Preheat an oven to 350°F-176°C. Take 12 muffins pans or a muffin tray; grease one by one with some coconut oil or butter. (You can also use coconut oil cooking spray to grease)
2. Heat the sausage with some olive oil in a skillet over medium stove flame. Break up sausage using a spatula while cooking.
3. Add the onion, pepper, spinach and oregano. Stir-cook until turns softened. Set aside.
4. Beat the eggs in a mixing bowl, add the pepper, salt and milk and combine well. Add the sausage mixture to the egg mixture.
5. Combine well until smooth batter is formed without any visible lumps.
6. Add the prepared batter evenly in the greased muffin pans or a tray; bake for 20 minutes or until turns golden brown. You can check by inserting a toothpick; when the bread is baked well, toothpick comes out clean.
7. Take out and allow to cool down on a wired rack for at least 10-20 minutes. Serve and enjoy.

NUTRITIONAL VALUES (PER SERVING):

Calories:142
F:11g C:4g fi:0g P:7g

Cranberry Spiced Muffins

Servings:
12

Preparation Time:
25-30 mins

Method:
Bake

INGREDIENTS:

1 ½ cup almond flour

½ cup coconut flour

1 teaspoon ground cinnamon

½ teaspoon ground ginger

¼ teaspoon salt

½ cup erythritol

3 teaspoons baking powder

½ cup coconut oil

1 cup unsweetened pumpkin puree

2 eggs

½ unsweetened dried cranberries

½ cup chopped pecans

DIRECTIONS:

1. Preheat an oven to 400ºF-204ºC. Take 12 muffins pans or a muffin tray; grease one by one with some coconut oil or butter. (You can also use coconut oil cooking spray to grease)
2. In a mixing bowl, combine the almond flour, coconut flour, sweetener, baking powder, cinnamon, ginger, and salt.
3. Beat the eggs in a mixing bowl; add the pumpkin, coconut oil, cranberries, and pecans.
4. Combine both mixtures with each other. Combine well until smooth batter is formed without any visible lumps.
5. Add the prepared batter evenly in the greased muffin pans or a tray; bake for 20-25 minutes or until turns golden brown. You can check by inserting a toothpick; when the bread is baked well, toothpick comes out clean.
6. Take out and allow to cool down on a wired rack for at least 10-20 minutes. Serve and enjoy.

NUTRITIONAL VALUES (PER SERVING):

Calories:128
F:21g C:10g fi:4g P:6g

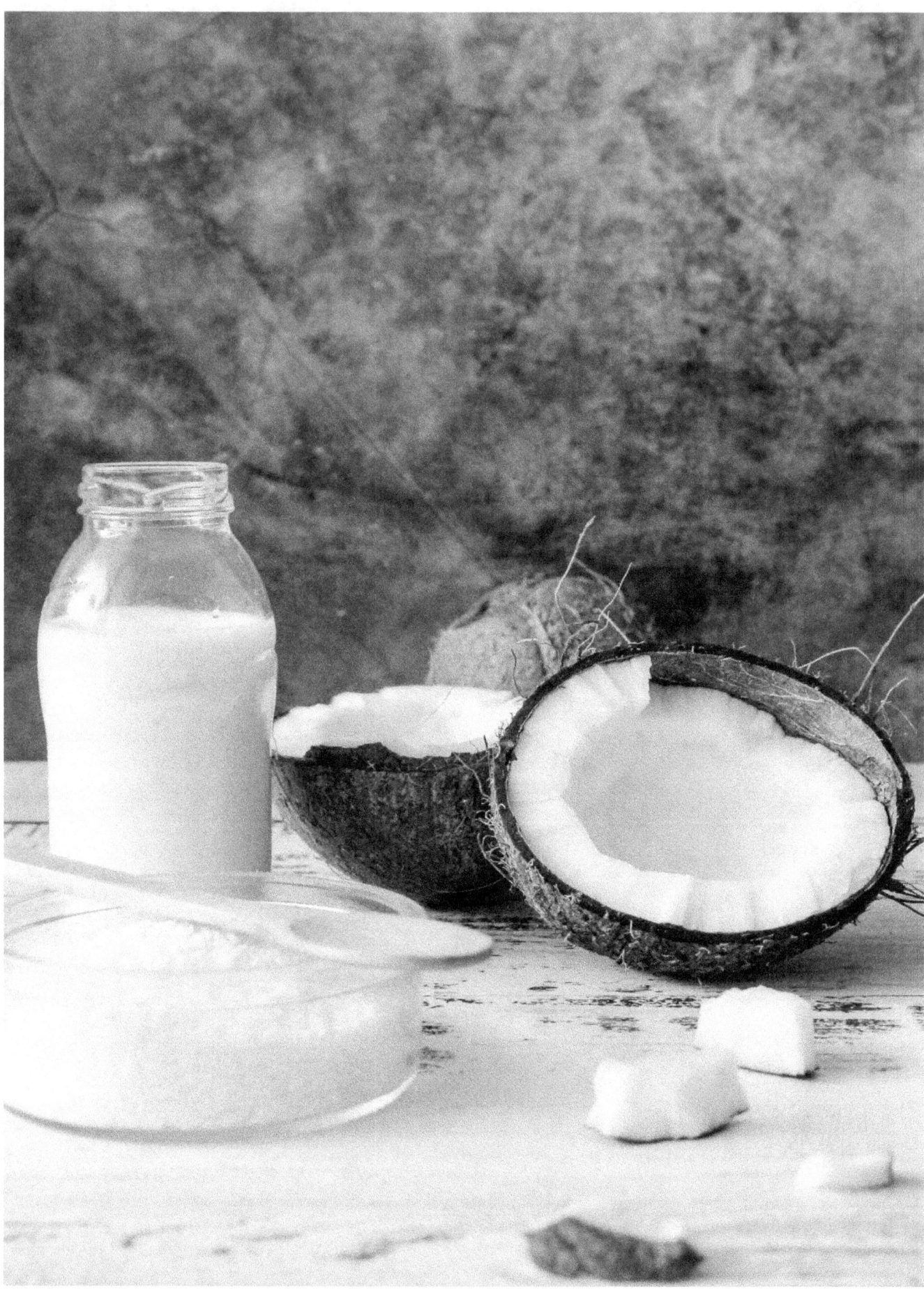

Coconut Craving Muffins

 **Servings:** 6-8

 **Preparation Time:** 25-30 mins

 **Method:** Bake

INGREDIENTS:

- ½ cup coconut flakes
- ¼ cup butter
- 3 eggs
- ¼ cup coconut flour
- 3 Tablespoon coconut milk
- ¼ cup erythritol
- Juice and grated zest of 1 lemon
- ½ teaspoon baking powder
- ½ teaspoon vanilla extract

DIRECTIONS:

1. Preheat an oven to 400°F-204°C. Take 6-8 muffins pans or a muffin tray; grease one by one with some coconut oil or butter. (You can also use coconut oil cooking spray to grease)
2. In a mixing bowl, whisk together the butter and erythritol until smooth. Mix in the eggs; whisk the mixture well.
3. Add the vanilla extract, lemon juice, lemon zest and coconut milk, mix well. Add the flour, coconut flakes and baking powder.
4. Combine well until smooth batter is formed without any visible lumps.
5. Add the prepared batter evenly in the greased muffin pans or a tray; bake for 20 minutes or until turns golden brown. You can check by inserting a toothpick; when the bread is baked well, toothpick comes out clean.
6. Take out and allow to cool down on a wired rack for at least 10-20 minutes. Serve and enjoy.

NUTRITIONAL VALUES (PER SERVING):

Calories: 251
F: 24g C: 9g fi: 3g P: 6g

Just Zucchini Muffins

Servings:
8-10

Preparation Time:
30-40 mins

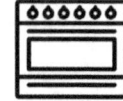

Method:
Bake

INGREDIENTS:

- 1 teaspoon baking powder
- 1 ½ cups zucchini, grated
- ¾ cup coconut flour
- 6 eggs
- ½ cup butter, melted
- 1 cup cheddar cheese, grated
- ½ teaspoon pepper
- ½ teaspoon salt
- 2 Tablespoons oregano, chopped finely

DIRECTIONS:

1. Preheat an oven to 350°F-176°C. Take 8-10 muffins pans or a muffin tray; grease one by one with some coconut oil or butter. (You can also use coconut oil cooking spray to grease)
2. In a mixing bowl, combine the zucchini, pepper, butter, and salt.
3. Whisk the eggs in another bowl, mix in the baking powder and oregano. Add the coconut flour and mix again. Add the cheese and combine well.
4. Combine both mixtures with each other. Combine well until smooth batter is formed without any visible lumps.
5. Add the prepared batter evenly in the greased muffin pans or a tray; bake for 25 minutes or until turns golden brown. You can check by inserting a toothpick; when the bread is baked well, toothpick comes out clean.
6. Take out and allow to cool down on a wired rack for at least 10-20 minutes. Serve and enjoy.

NUTRITIONAL VALUES (PER SERVING):

Calories:182
F:15g C:1g Fi:0g P:7g

Classic Keto Muffins

Servings:
6

Preparation Time:
20-25 mins

Method:
Bake

INGREDIENTS:

6 egg

3 Tablespoons coconut flour

1 ½ teaspoons baking powder

Salt to taste

Liquid Stevia to taste (optional)

DIRECTIONS:

1. Preheat an oven to 400°F-204°C. Take 6 muffins pans or a muffin tray; grease one by one with some coconut oil or butter. (You can also use coconut oil cooking spray to grease)
2. Whisk all ingredients in a mixing bowl to combine well, until no lumps visible.
3. Add the prepared batter evenly in the greased muffin pans or a tray; bake for 10-12 minutes or until turns golden brown. You can check by inserting a toothpick; when the bread is baked well, toothpick comes out clean.
4. Take out and allow to cool down on a wired rack for at least 10-20 minutes. Serve and enjoy.

NUTRITIONAL VALUES (PER SERVING):

Calories: 139
F:8g C:4g fi:0.5g P:7g

Hazelnut Muffins

Servings:
12

Preparation Time:
30-35 mins

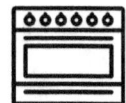

Method:
Bake

INGREDIENTS:

2 cups hazelnuts

5 eggs, beaten

10-15 drops (or to taste) liquid Stevia

Ground cinnamon to taste

DIRECTIONS:

1. Preheat an oven to 350°F-176°C. Take 12 muffins pans or a muffin tray; grease one by one with some coconut oil or butter. (You can also use coconut oil cooking spray to grease)
2. Add the hazelnuts in a blender or food processor. Blend to form a flour.
3. Beat the eggs and add it with the hazelnut flour in a mixing bowl. Mix thoroughly.
4. Add the stevia and cinnamon; combine well.
5. Add the prepared batter evenly in the greased muffin pans or a tray; bake for 25 minutes or until turns golden brown. You can check by inserting a toothpick; when the bread is baked well, toothpick comes out clean.
6. Take out and allow to cool down on a wired rack for at least 10-20 minutes. Serve and enjoy.

NUTRITIONAL VALUES (PER SERVING):

Calories: 112
F: 10g C: 4g fi: 1g P: 6g

Lemon Cream Muffins

Servings:
12

Preparation Time:
25-30 mins

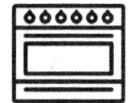

Method:
Bake

INGREDIENTS:

- ¾ cup almond flour
- 1/3 cup Erythritol
- 3 large eggs
- Zest of 2 lemons
- ¼ cup golden flaxseed meal
- ¼ cup heavy cream
- ¼ cup salted butter (melted)
- 1 teaspoon baking powder
- 1 teaspoon vanilla extract
- 3 Tablespoons lemon juice
- 2 Tablespoons poppy seeds
- 20-25 drops liquid Stevia

DIRECTIONS:

1. Preheat an oven to 350ºF-176ºC. Take 12 muffins pans or a muffin tray; grease one by one with some coconut oil or butter. (You can also use coconut oil cooking spray to grease)
2. Combine the almond flour, flaxseed meal, Erythritol and poppy seeds in a mixing bowl.
3. Beat the eggs in another mixing bowl, mix in the heavy cream and butter. Add the baking powder, vanilla, Stevia, lemon zest and lemon juice; combine again.
4. Combine both mixtures with each other. Combine well until smooth batter is formed without any visible lumps.
5. Add the prepared batter evenly in the greased muffin pans or a tray; bake for 20 minutes or until turns golden brown. You can check by inserting a toothpick; when the bread is baked well, toothpick comes out clean.
6. Take out and allow to cool down on a wired rack for at least 10-20 minutes. Serve and enjoy.

NUTRITIONAL VALUES (PER SERVING):

Calories:97
F:12g C:3g Fi:0g P:4g

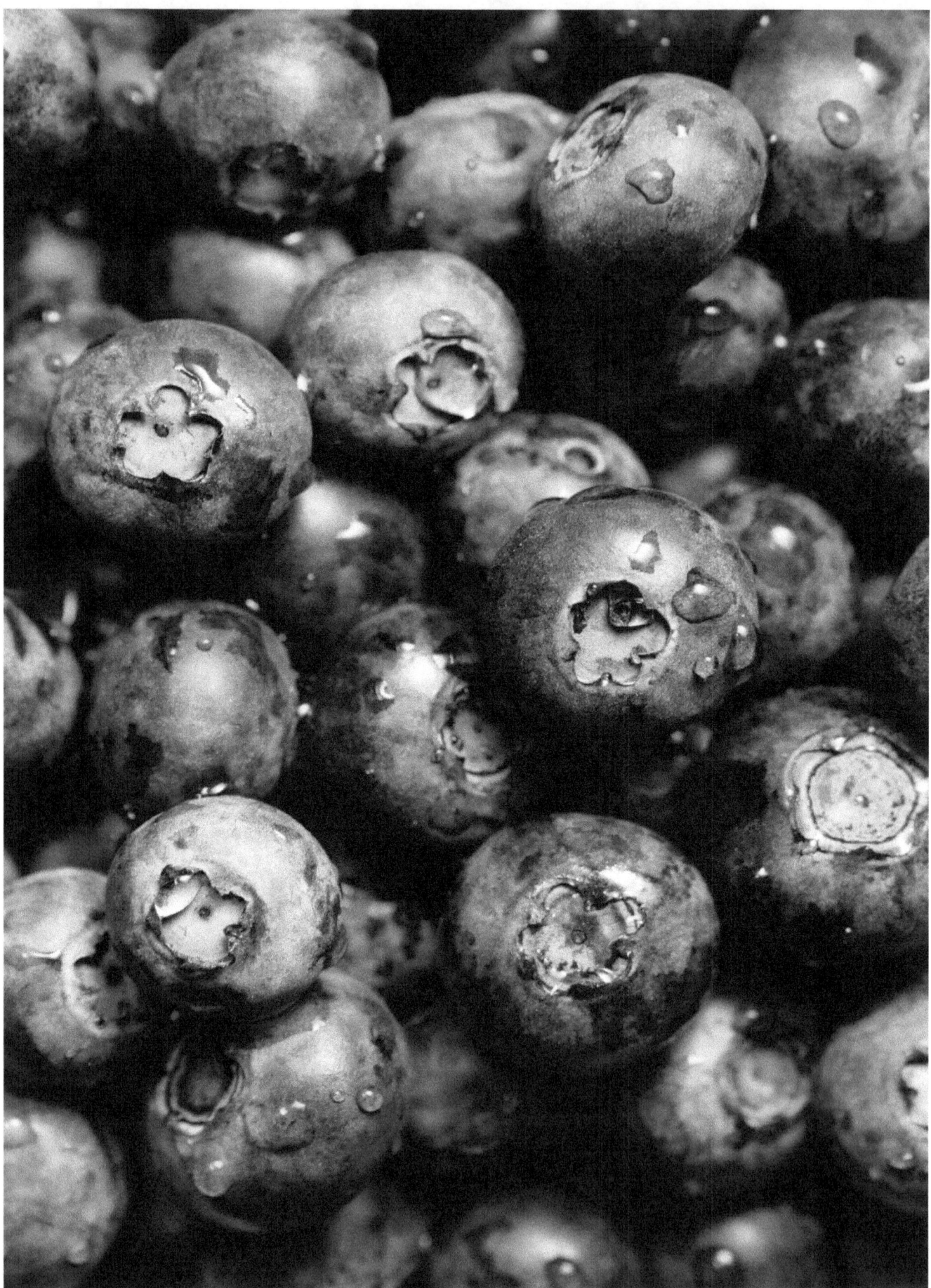

Blueberry Keto Muffins

Servings:
6

Preparation Time:
30-40 mins

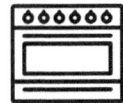

Method:
Bake

INGREDIENTS:

1 teaspoon baking powder

¼ cup warm water

¼ cup coconut flour

½ cup almond flour

¼ cup blueberries

3 eggs

2 Tablespoons butter, melted

¼ teaspoon salt

¼ teaspoon liquid Stevia

½ teaspoon lemon extract

2 Tablespoons powdered erythritol

DIRECTIONS:

1. Preheat an oven to 350ºF-176ºC. Take 6 muffins pans or a muffin tray; grease one by one with some coconut oil or butter. (You can also use coconut oil cooking spray to grease)
2. Mix the almond flour, coconut flour, baking powder and salt in a mixing bowl. In another bowl, whisk the eggs, butter, water, erythritol, stevia and lemon extract.
3. Combine both mixtures with each other. Combine well until smooth batter is formed without any visible lumps. Mix in the blueberries.
4. Add the prepared batter evenly in the greased muffin pans or a tray; bake for 20-25 minutes or until turns golden brown. You can check by inserting a toothpick; when the bread is baked well, toothpick comes out clean.
5. Take out and allow to cool down on a wired rack for at least 10-20 minutes. Serve and enjoy.

NUTRITIONAL VALUES (PER SERVING):

Calories:148
F:12g C:6g Fi:2g P:6g

Cinnamon Roll Muffins

Servings:
3-4

Preparation Time:
25-30 mins

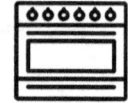

Method:
Bake

INGREDIENTS:

2 eggs

7 ounces cottage cheese

¼ teaspoon liquid Stevia

½ cup coconut flour

⅓ teaspoon baking powder

Salt to taste (optional)

Filling:

¼ teaspoon liquid Stevia

2 teaspoon cinnamon

1 ounce erythritol

2 Tablespoons butter, melted

DIRECTIONS:

1. Preheat an oven to 350°F-176°C. Prepare a baking sheet by lining it with a parchment paper. Grease it with some coconut oil or butter. (You can also use coconut oil cooking spray to grease)
2. In a mixing bowl, beat the eggs; mix in the cottage cheese, stevia and erythritol. In another bowl, combine the coconut flour and baking powder.
3. Combine both mixtures with each other. Combine well until smooth batter is formed without any visible lumps.
4. Wrap the prepared dough with a plastic sheet. Start rolling it into ¼ inch thin layer. Remove the plastic sheet and brush melted butter over it and top with the cinnamon.
5. Roll the layer into circular shape and cut into 8 pieces. Place over baking sheet; bake for 15 minutes or until turns golden brown.
6. Take out the baking sheet and allow it to cool down on a wired rack for at least 10-20 minutes.
7. Serve and enjoy!

NUTRITIONAL VALUES (PER SERVING):

Calories:114
F:7g C:1g Fi:0g P:7g

CHAPTER 4
KETO BUNS

Almond Hamburger Buns

Servings:
6

Preparation Time:
70-80 mins

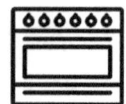

Method:
Bake

INGREDIENTS:

1 cup water (boiling)

3 egg whites

1 ¼ cups almond flour

5 Tablespoons psyllium husk powder (ground)

2 teaspoons baking powder

2 teaspoons apple cider vinegar

1 teaspoon sea salt

DIRECTIONS:

1. Preheat an oven to 350°F-176°C. Prepare a baking sheet by lining it with a parchment paper. Grease it with some coconut oil or butter. (You can also use coconut oil cooking spray to grease)
2. Beat the eggs in a mixing bowl. Mix in the vinegar.
3. In a mixing bowl, combine all the dry ingredients.
4. Combine both mixtures with each other; add the boiling water. Combine well until a well-mixed dough is formed.
5. Divide the dough into six small rounds.
6. Place the rounds over the lined baking sheet. Using hands or spoon, give them a hamburger bun shape (it will create a dome shaped top) and bake for 55-60 minutes or until turns light brown.
7. Take out and allow it to cool down on a wired rack for at least 15-20 minutes.
8. Serve and enjoy!

NUTRITIONAL VALUES (PER SERVING):

Calories: 81
F:9g C:2g Fi:0g P:3g

Classic Sesame Buns

Servings:
8-10

Preparation Time:
50-60 mins

Method:
Bake

INGREDIENTS:

Dry ingredients:

½ cup coconut flour

½ cup flax meal

1 ½ cups almond flour

⅔ cup psyllium husks

2 teaspoons garlic powder

2 teaspoons onion powder

1 teaspoon baking soda

5 Tablespoons sesame seeds

2 teaspoons cream of tartar

1 teaspoon salt

Wet ingredients:

2 large eggs

6 large egg whites

2 cups water (boiling)

DIRECTIONS:

1. Preheat an oven to 350°F-176°C. Prepare a baking sheet by lining it with a parchment paper. Grease it with some coconut oil or butter. (You can also use coconut oil cooking spray to grease)
2. Beat the eggs and egg whites in a mixing bowl.
3. In a mixing bowl, combine all the dry ingredients except the seeds.
4. Combine both mixtures with each other; add boiling water. Combine well until a well-mixed dough is formed.
5. Divide the dough into small rounds.
6. Place the rounds over the lined baking sheet. Using hands or spoon, give them a bun shape (it will create a dome shaped top).
7. Sprinkle with the sesame seeds, gently press, and bake for 45 minutes or until turns light brown.
8. Take out and allow it to cool down on a wired rack for at least 15-20 minutes.
9. Serve and enjoy!

NUTRITIONAL VALUES (PER SERVING):

Calories:186
F:15g C:8g Fi:2g P:10g

Cheesy Hamburger Buns

Servings:
5-6

Preparation Time:
40-45 mins

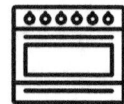

Method:
Bake

INGREDIENTS:

1 ½ cup mozzarella cheese, grated

1 tablespoon baking powder

2 ounce cream cheese

1 ¼ cup almond flour

1 egg

DIRECTIONS:

1. Preheat an oven to 400°F-204°C. Prepare a baking sheet by lining it with a parchment paper. Grease it with some coconut oil or butter. (You can also use coconut oil cooking spray to grease)
2. In a heatproof bowl, add the mozzarella cheese and cream cheese. Microwave until melts completely.
3. Beat the eggs in a mixing bowl. Add the cheese mix and combine.
4. In a mixing bowl, combine all the dry ingredients.
5. Combine both mixtures with each other. Combine well until a well-mixed dough is formed.
6. Divide the dough into 5-6 small rounds.
7. Place the rounds over the lined baking sheet. Using hands or spoon, give them a hamburger bun shape (it will create a dome shaped top) and bake for 10-12 minutes or until turns light brown.
8. Take out and allow it to cool down on a wired rack for at least 15-20 minutes.
9. Serve and enjoy!

NUTRITIONAL VALUES (PER SERVING):

Calories:283
F:24g C:4g fi:1g P:14g

Garlic Keto Buns

Servings:
8-10

Preparation Time:
60-70 mins

Method:
Bake

INGREDIENTS:

Dry ingredients:

- ⅔ cup flax meal
- ⅓ cup psyllium husk powder
- 1 ¼ cups sesame seed flour
- ⅔ cup coconut flour
- 2 teaspoons cream of tartar
- 2 teaspoons garlic powder
- 2 teaspoons onion powder
- 5 Tablespoons sesame seeds
- 1 teaspoon salt
- 1 teaspoon baking soda

Wet ingredients:

- 2 large eggs
- 6 large egg whites
- 2 ½ cups water (boiling)

DIRECTIONS:

1. Preheat an oven to 350°F-176°C. Prepare a baking sheet by lining it with a parchment paper. Grease it with some coconut oil or butter. (You can also use coconut oil cooking spray to grease)
2. Beat the eggs and egg whites in a mixing bowl
3. In a mixing bowl, combine all the dry ingredients. Except the sesame seeds.
4. Combine both mixtures with each other; add boiling water. Combine well until a well-mixed dough is formed.
5. Divide the dough into small rounds.
6. Place the rounds over the lined baking sheet. Using hands or spoon, give them a bun shape (it will create a dome shaped top).
7. Sprinkle with the sesame seeds, gently press, and bake for 55-60 minutes or until turns light brown.
8. Take out and allow it to cool down on a wired rack for at least 15-20 minutes.
9. Serve and enjoy!

NUTRITIONAL VALUES (PER SERVING):

Calories:183
F:12g C:7g fi:5g P:12g

Pumpkin Keto Buns

Servings:
10-12

Preparation Time:
60-70 mins

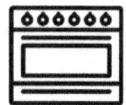

Method:
Bake

INGREDIENTS:

- 1 cup hot water
- ½ cup psyllium powder
- 8 egg whites
- 1 cup coconut flour
- ½ cup pumpkin seeds
- 1 cup sesame seeds
- 1 Tablespoon sea salt
- 1 Tablespoon baking powder

DIRECTIONS:

1. Preheat an oven to 350°F-176°C. Prepare a baking sheet by lining it with a parchment paper. Grease it with some coconut oil or butter. (You can also use coconut oil cooking spray to grease)
2. Beat the egg whites in a mixing bowl.
3. In a mixing bowl, combine all the dry ingredients (use ½ cup sesame seeds).
4. Combine both mixtures with each other; add boiling water. Combine well until a well-mixed dough is formed.
5. Divide the dough into small rounds.
6. Place the rounds over the lined baking sheet. Using hands or spoon, give them a bun shape (it will create a dome shaped top).
7. Sprinkle the sesame seeds on top, gently press, and bake for 50 minutes or until turns light brown.
8. Take out and allow it to cool down on a wired rack for at least 15-20 minutes.
9. Serve and enjoy!

NUTRITIONAL VALUES (PER SERVING):

Calories:134
F:13g C:9g Fi:7g P:6g

Everyday Breakfast Buns

Servings:
6

Preparation Time:
30-40 mins

Method:
Bake

INGREDIENTS:

5 tablespoons butter, melted

2 large eggs

¾ cup almond flour

1 ½ Tablespoons baking powder

DIRECTIONS:

1. Preheat an oven to 350°F-176°C. Prepare a baking sheet by lining it with a parchment paper. Grease it with some coconut oil or butter. (You can also use coconut oil cooking spray to grease)
2. Combine the almond flour and baking powder in a mixing bowl. Beat the eggs in another bowl; mix in the butter.
3. Combine both mixtures with each other. Combine well until a well-mixed dough is formed.
4. Divide the dough into six small rounds.
5. Place the rounds over the lined baking sheet. Using hands or spoon, give them a bun shape (it will create a dome shaped top) and bake for 15 minutes or until turns light brown.
6. Take out and allow it to cool down on a wired rack for at least 15-20 minutes.
7. Serve and enjoy!

NUTRITIONAL VALUES (PER SERVING):

Calories:153
F:17g C:4g Fi:1g P:5g

Mix Seed Mystery Bagels

Servings:
6

Preparation Time:
60-70 mins

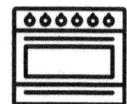

Method:
Bake

INGREDIENTS:

½ cup sesame seeds

½ cup pumpkin seeds

¼ cup psyllium husk

½ cup hemp hearts

1 cup coconut flour

1 teaspoon salt

1 Tablespoon baking powder

6 egg whites

1 cup boiling water

DIRECTIONS:

1. Preheat an oven to 350°F-176°C. Prepare a baking sheet by lining it with a parchment paper. Grease it with some coconut oil or butter. (You can also use coconut oil cooking spray to grease)
2. In a mixing bowl, beat the egg whites. Add the water and combine well. In another mixing bowl, combine the remaining ingredients except the sesame seeds.
3. Combine both mixtures with each other. Combine well until a well-mixed dough is formed.
4. Divide the dough into 6 pieces. Roll them using a rolling pin and joint ends to create a bagel shape. Top with the sesame seeds and gently press.
5. Place them over the lined baking sheet; bake for 55-60 minutes or until turns light brown.
6. Take out and allow it to cool down on a wired rack for at least 15-20 minutes.
7. Serve and enjoy!

NUTRITIONAL VALUES (PER SERVING):

Calories:197
F:15g C:9g fi:4g P:11g

Cheesy Bagels

Servings:
5-6

Preparation Time:
30-40 mins

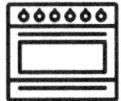

Method:
Bake

INGREDIENTS:

2 ½ cups mozzarella cheese (shredded)

1 ½ cups almond flour

2 large eggs, beaten

2 ounces cream cheese (cubed)

1 Tablespoon baking powder

DIRECTIONS:

1. Preheat an oven to 400°F-204°C. Prepare a baking sheet by lining it with a parchment paper. Grease it with some coconut oil or butter. (You can also use coconut oil cooking spray to grease)
2. Combine the almond flour and baking powder in a mixing bowl. Combine the mozzarella and cream cheese in a heatproof bowl. Microwave until melts completely.
3. Combine both mixtures with each other. Combine well until a well-mixed dough is formed.
4. Divide the dough into 6 pieces. Roll them using a rolling pin and joint ends to create a bagel shape. Top with the sesame seeds and gently press.
5. Place them over the lined baking sheet; bake for 10-12 minutes or until turns light brown.
6. Take out and allow it to cool down on a wired rack for at least 15-20 minutes.
7. Serve and enjoy!

NUTRITIONAL VALUES (PER SERVING):

Calories: 324
F:26g C:8g Fi:4g P:20g

CHAPTER 5
KETO BREADS ROLLS

Classic Dinner Rolls

Servings:
10

Preparation Time:
30-35 mins

Method:
Bake

INGREDIENTS:

½ cup coconut flour

4 Tablespoons butter (melted)

2 Tablespoons psyllium husk powder

¼ teaspoon salt

½ teaspoon baking powder

4 large eggs

¾ cup water

DIRECTIONS:

1. Preheat an oven to 350ºF-176ºC. Prepare a baking sheet by lining it with a parchment paper. Grease it with some coconut oil or butter. (You can also use coconut oil cooking spray to grease)
2. Beat the eggs in a mixing bowl. Mix in the butter and water. In a mixing bowl, combine all the dry ingredients.
3. Combine both mixtures with each other. Combine well until a well-mixed dough is formed. Prepare small sized molds from the dough. Using hands, shape them into 10 rolls.
4. Place the rolls over the lined baking sheet, and bake for 35 minutes or until turns light brown.
5. Take out and allow it to cool down on a wired rack for at least 15-20 minutes.
6. Serve and enjoy!

NUTRITIONAL VALUES (PER SERVING):

Calories:93
F:8g C:6g Fi:2g P:3g

Zucchini Bread Rolls

Servings:
10

Preparation Time:
60-70 mins

Method:
Bake

INGREDIENTS:

4 pastured eggs

2 Tablespoons avocado oil

2 Tablespoons psyllium husk powder

8 Tablespoons coconut flour

1 zucchini, peeled and finely grated

3 teaspoon baking powder

¼ cup water

1 Tablespoon dried basil

½ teaspoon sea salt

2 Tablespoons apple cider vinegar

DIRECTIONS:

1. Preheat an oven to 350°F-176°C. Prepare a baking sheet by lining it with a parchment paper. Grease it with some coconut oil or butter. (You can also use coconut oil cooking spray to grease)
2. In a mixing bowl, combine the psyllium husk, salt, herbs, flour and baking powder. Combine well.
3. Beat the eggs in a mixing bowl; add remaining ingredients and combine well.
4. Combine both mixtures with each other. Combine well until a well-mixed dough is formed. Prepare small sized molds from the dough. Using hands, shape them into rolls.
5. Place the rolls over the lined baking sheet, and bake for 45 minutes or until turns light brown.
6. Take out and allow it to cool down on a wired rack for at least 15-20 minutes.
7. Serve and enjoy!

NUTRITIONAL VALUES (PER SERVING):

Calories: 91
F:9g C:5g Fi:3g P:2g

Round Bread Rolls

Servings:
7

Preparation Time:
40-50 mins

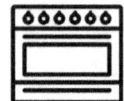

Method:
Bake

INGREDIENTS:

3 Tablespoons lukewarm water

1 Tablespoon active dry yeast

¼ cup coconut cream

2 ½ Tablespoons apple cider vinegar

Liquid Stevia to taste

2 ¼ cups almond flour

2 teaspoons salt

2 ½ teaspoons baking powder

6 Tablespoons golden flax seeds, ground

1 Tablespoon psyllium husk powder

3 large eggs

2 Tablespoons coconut oil

DIRECTIONS:

1. Preheat an oven to 400°F-204°C. Prepare a baking sheet by lining it with a parchment paper. Grease it with some coconut oil or butter. (You can also use coconut oil cooking spray to grease)
2. Combine the coconut cream, 2 teaspoon cider vinegar, water and Stevia in a mixing bowl. Mix in the yeast and set aside for 10-15 minutes.
3. In another bowl, combine the almond flour, baking powder, flax seeds, salt, and psyllium powder.
4. Beat eggs in a bowl; mix in the coconut oil, yeast mixture.
5. Combine both mixtures with each other. Combine well until a well-mixed dough is formed. Prepare 7 molds from the dough. Using hands, shape them into round rolls. Set aside for 1 hour to rise.
6. Place the rolls over the lined baking sheet, and bake for 15-20 minutes or until turns light brown.
7. Take out and allow it to cool down on a wired rack for at least 15-20 minutes.
8. Serve and enjoy!

NUTRITIONAL VALUES (PER SERVING):

Calories:234
F:18g C:7g fi:2g P:14g

Mozzarella Bread Rolls

Servings:
10-12

Preparation Time:
30-40 mins

Method:
Bake

INGREDIENTS:

- 4 Tablespoons baking powder
- 4 large eggs
- 1 ⅓ cups almond flour
- 1 Tablespoons butter, unsalted
- 8 ounces cream cheese
- 3 cups mozzarella cheese, shredded

DIRECTIONS:

1. Preheat an oven to 400°F-204°C. Prepare a baking sheet by lining it with a parchment paper. Grease it with some coconut oil or butter. (You can also use coconut oil cooking spray to grease)
2. In a heatproof bowl, add the mozzarella and cream cheese. Microwave until melts completely.
3. Beat the eggs in a mixing bowl. Mix in the cheese mixture.
4. In a mixing bowl, combine all the almond flour and baking powder.
5. Combine both mixtures with each other. Combine well until a well-mixed dough is formed. Set aside for 20 minutes.
6. Prepare 24 molds from the dough. Using hands, shape them into rolls; brush them with melted butter.
7. Place the rolls over the lined baking sheet, and bake for 20-25 minutes or until turns light brown.
8. Take out and allow it to cool down on a wired rack for at least 15-20 minutes.
9. Serve and enjoy!

NUTRITIONAL VALUES (PER SERVING):

Calories: 175
F:16g C:4g Fi:2g P:11g

Classic Oregano Pizza Crust

Servings:
1 crust (8 slices)

Preparation Time:
35-40 mins

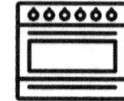

Method:
Bake

INGREDIENTS:

½ cup parmesan cheese grated

1 ½ cups almond flour

1 tablespoon olive oil

½ teaspoon baking powder

1 tablespoon whole psyllium husks or flax meal

½ teaspoon basil, chopped

½ teaspoon oregano

2 large eggs

½ teaspoon garlic powder

2 tablespoons water, more if required

DIRECTIONS:

1. Preheat an oven to 375ºF-190ºC. Prepare two parchment papers by greasing with some coconut oil or butter. (You can also use coconut oil cooking spray to grease). Also grease a pizza pan with some butter or coconut oil.
2. Beat the eggs in a mixing bowl. Mix in the olive oil. In a mixing bowl, combine all the dry ingredients.
3. Combine both mixtures with each other. Combine well until a well-mixed dough is formed.
4. Place the prepared dough between two greased papers. Using a rolling pin, roll out the dough into an even round shape.
5. Add the crust in the greased pan, remove top paper and fold the edges of the crust with wet fingertips. Bake for 20-25 until the crust becomes light brown.
6. Take it out and cool down for 10-15 minutes. The crust is ready to be used to preparing pizza with keto friendly ingredients.

NUTRITIONAL VALUES (PER SERVING):

Calories:173
F:14g C:6g fi:3g P:8g

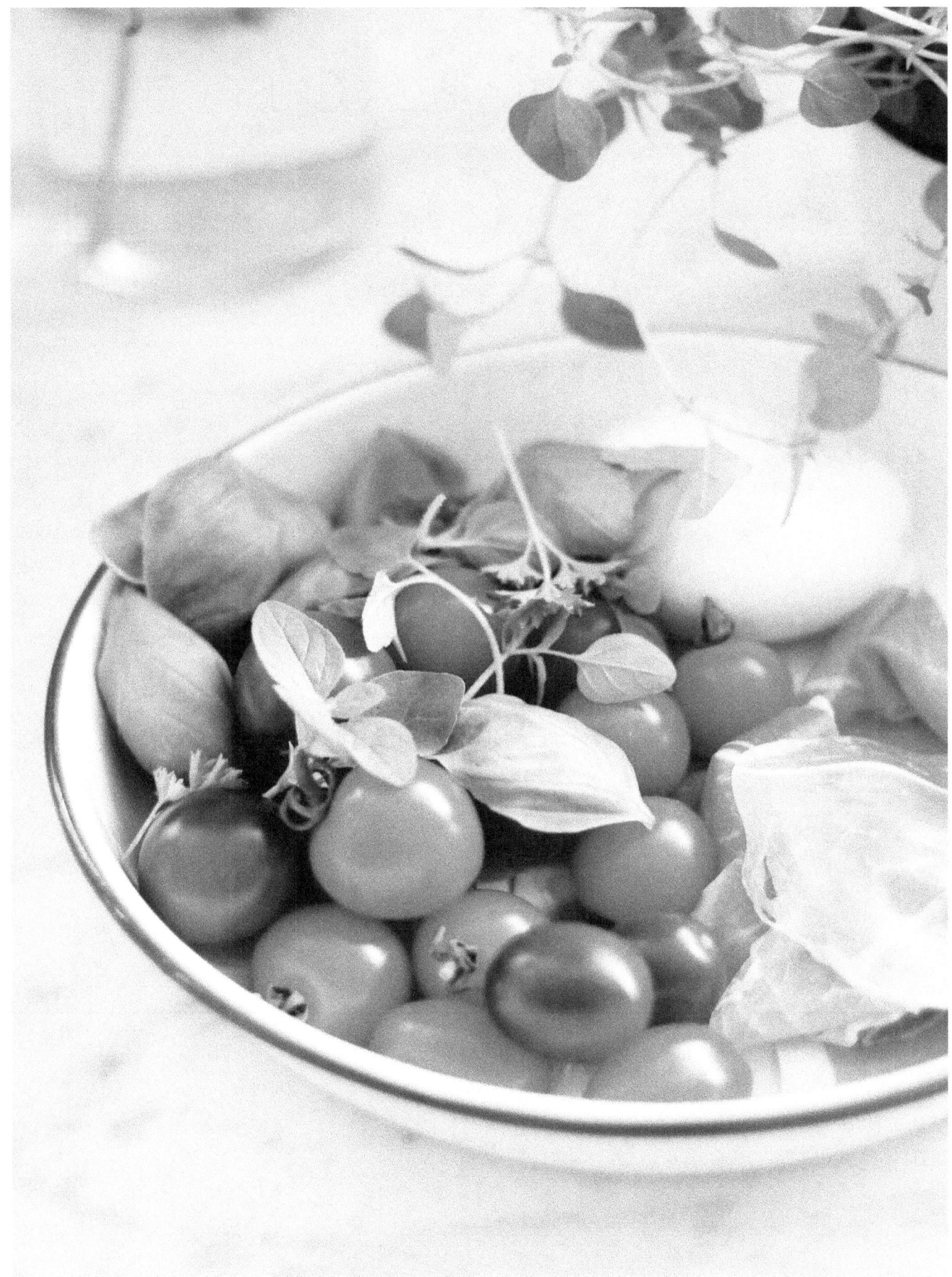

Mozzarella Pizza Crust

Servings:
1 crust (6-8 slices)

Preparation Time:
20 mins

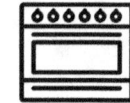

Method:
Bake

INGREDIENTS:

5 Tablespoons butter, melted

2 teaspoon baking powder

6 ounces mozzarella cheese, shredded

1 large egg

¼ cup coconut flour

½ cup blanched almond flour

¼ teaspoon salt

½ teaspoon garlic powder

DIRECTIONS:

1. Preheat an oven to 350°F-176°C. Prepare two parchment papers by greasing with some coconut oil or butter. (You can also use coconut oil cooking spray to grease). Also grease a pizza pan with some butter or coconut oil.
2. Beat the eggs in a mixing bowl. Mix in the butter. In a mixing bowl, combine all the dry ingredients.
3. Combine both mixtures with each other. Combine well until a well-mixed dough is formed.
4. Place the prepared dough between two greased papers. Using a rolling pin, roll out the dough into an even round shape.
5. Add the crust in the greased pan, remove top paper and fold the edges of the crust with wet fingertips. Bake for 10-15 until the crust becomes light brown.
6. Take it out and cool down for 10-15 minutes. The crust is ready to be used to preparing pizza with keto friendly ingredients.

NUTRITIONAL VALUES (PER SERVING):

Calories: 217
F:19g C:6g Fi:2g P:9g

CHAPTER 6
KETO BREADSTICKS

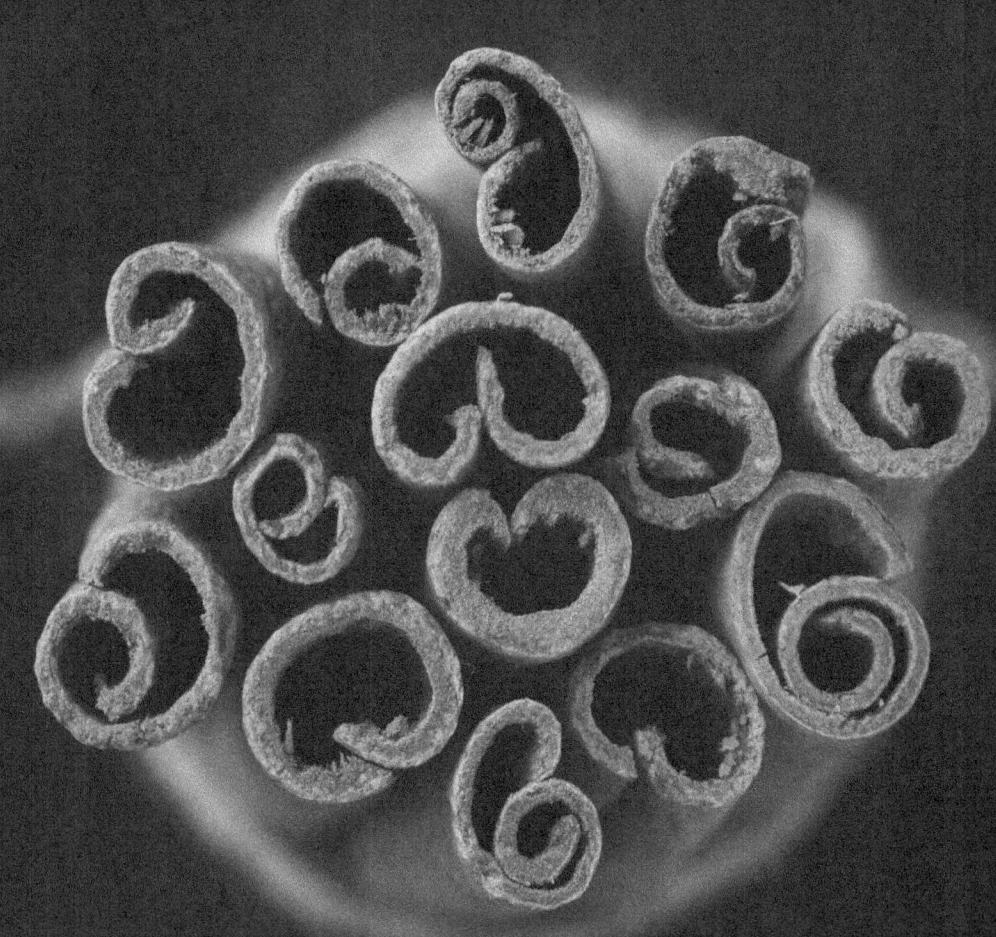

Aromatic Cinnamon Breadsticks

Servings:
8-10

Preparation Time:
30-40 mins

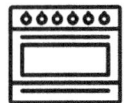

Method:
Bake

INGREDIENTS:

¾ cup almond flour

3 Tablespoons cream cheese

1 Tablespoon psyllium husk powder

1 large egg

2 cups mozzarella cheese

1 teaspoon baking powder

Flavorings:

3 Tablespoons butter

2 Tablespoons cinnamon

6 Tablespoons Stevia granular

DIRECTIONS:

1. Preheat an oven to 400°F-204°C. Prepare a baking sheet by lining it with a parchment paper. Grease it with some coconut oil or butter. (You can also use coconut oil cooking spray to grease)
2. Mix the egg and cream cheese in mixing bowl.
3. Mix the almond flour, psyllium husk powder and baking powder in another mixing bowl.
4. Microwave the mozzarella cheese until melts completely. Add it with the egg mixture and combine.
5. Combine both mixtures with each other. Combine well until a well-combined dough is formed without any visible lumps.
6. Place the prepared breadstick dough over a lined baking sheet. Using your hands, press it to shape into a rectangle. Take a pizza cutter and make cuts to prepare unbaked breadsticks.
7. Combine all the flavoring ingredients. Top each breadsticks evenly with the flavor mixture.
8. Bake for 15 minutes or until turns crisp to your satisfaction.
9. Take it out and allow to cool down on a wired rack for at least 10-20 minutes. Serve and enjoy.

NUTRITIONAL VALUES (PER SERVING):

Calories: 263
F: 20g C: 6g Fi: 3g P: 13g

Italian Style Cheesy Breadsticks

Servings:
10-12

Preparation Time:
30-35 mins

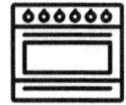

Method:
Bake

INGREDIENTS:

¾ cup almond flour

1 Tablespoon psyllium husk powder

2 cups shredded mozzarella cheese

1 egg (lightly beaten)

3 Tablespoons cream cheese

1 Tablespoon butter, melted

2 teaspoons Italian herb blend (dried)

1 teaspoon ground black pepper

DIRECTIONS:

1. Preheat an oven to 400ºF-204ºC. Prepare a baking sheet by lining it with a parchment paper. Grease it with some coconut oil or butter. (You can also use coconut oil cooking spray to grease)
2. In a mixing bowl, beat the egg and cream cheese. In another bowl, mix the almond flour, psyllium husk powder, and baking powder.
3. In a heatproof bowl, add the mozzarella cheese and cream cheese. Microwave until melts completely. Add it to the egg mixture and combine well.
4. Combine both mixtures with each other. Combine well until a well-combined dough is formed without any visible lumps.
5. Place the prepared breadstick dough over a lined baking sheet. Using your hands, press it to shape into a rectangle. Take a pizza cutter and make cuts to prepare unbaked breadsticks.
6. Sprinkle each breadsticks evenly with Italian herb blend and pepper. Bake for 15 minutes or until turns crisp to your satisfaction.
7. Take it out and allow to cool down on a wired rack for at least 10-20 minutes. Serve and enjoy.

NUTRITIONAL VALUES (PER SERVING):

Calories:128
F:9g C:3g Fi:0g P:7g

Coconut Cheese Breadsticks

Servings:
8

Preparation Time:
30-40 mins

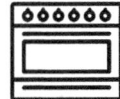

Method:
Bake

INGREDIENTS:

1 ⅓ cups mozzarella cheese (shredded)

½ cup parmesan cheese (shredded)

1/3 cup coconut flour

4 eggs

1 ounce cream cheese

4 ½ Tablespoons butter, melted

½ teaspoon garlic powder

¼ teaspoon baking powder

1 teaspoon Italian seasoning

¼ teaspoon salt

Toppings:

¼ cup parmesan cheese (shredded)

2 cups mozzarella cheese (shredded)

½ teaspoon Italian seasoning

DIRECTIONS:

1. Preheat an oven to 400°F-204°C. Prepare a baking sheet by lining it with a parchment paper. Grease it with some coconut oil or butter. (You can also use coconut oil cooking spray to grease)
2. Combine the eggs, cream cheese, butter and salt in a mixing bowl.
3. Add the coconut flour, baking powder, Italian seasoning and garlic powder in another mixing bowl. Add the mozzarella and parmesan cheese to the mixture.
4. Combine both mixtures with each other. Combine well until a well-combined dough is formed without any visible lumps.
5. Place the prepared breadstick dough over a lined baking sheet. Using your hands, press it to shape into a rectangle. Take a pizza cutter and make cuts to prepare unbaked breadsticks.
6. Sprinkle each breadsticks evenly with topping ingredients.
7. Bake for 15 minutes or until turns crisp to your satisfaction.
8. Take it out and allow to cool down on a wired rack for at least 10-20 minutes. Serve and enjoy.

NUTRITIONAL VALUES (PER SERVING):

Calories:357
F:26g C:7g fi:2g P:21g

Cheesy Garlic Breadsticks

Servings:
10

Preparation Time:
30-40 mins

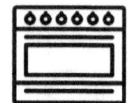
Method:
Bake

INGREDIENTS:

1 ¾ cups grated mozzarella cheese

¾ cups blanched almond flour

1 medium egg, room temperature

1 teaspoon baking soda

2 Tablespoons cream cheese

1 Tablespoon garlic, minced

¼ teaspoon salt

¼ cup shredded parmesan cheese

DIRECTIONS:

1. Preheat an oven to 425°F-232°C. Prepare a baking sheet by lining it with a parchment paper. Grease it with some coconut oil or butter. (You can also use coconut oil cooking spray to grease)
2. Combine the mozzarella and cream cheese in a heat-safe bowl. Microwave until melts completely. Stir in the egg, almond flour, garlic, baking soda, and salt.
3. Combine well until a well-combined dough is formed without any visible lumps.
4. Place the prepared breadstick dough over a lined baking sheet. Using your hands, press it to shape into a rectangle. Take a pizza cutter and make cuts to prepare unbaked breadsticks.
5. Sprinkle each breadsticks evenly with Parmesan cheese.
6. Bake for 15 minutes or until turns crisp to your satisfaction.
7. Take it out and allow to cool down on a wired rack for at least 10-20 minutes. Serve and enjoy.

NUTRITIONAL VALUES (PER SERVING):

Calories:102
F:8g C:1g Fi:0g P:7g

Seeded Keto Breadsticks

Servings:
10-12

Preparation Time:
20 mins

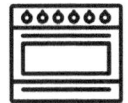
Method:
Bake

INGREDIENTS:

¾ cup flax meal

¼ cup coconut flour

1 cup almond flour

1 cup water (lukewarm)

2 Tablespoons psyllium husks powder

2 Tablespoons chia seeds (ground)

1 teaspoon salt

Toppings:

4 Tablespoons parmesan cheese (grated)

1 teaspoon sea salt (coarse)

2 large egg yolks

DIRECTIONS:

1. Preheat an oven to 350ºF-176ºC. Prepare a baking sheet by lining it with a parchment paper. Grease it with some coconut oil or butter. (You can also use coconut oil cooking spray to grease)
2. Combine the almond flour, flax meal, coconut flour and psyllium husks in a mixing bowl. Add the chia seeds and water. Combine well until a well-combined dough is formed without any visible lumps.
3. Place the prepared breadstick dough over a lined baking sheet. Using your hands, press it to shape into a rectangle. Take a pizza cutter and make cuts to prepare unbaked breadsticks.
4. Brush with the egg yolks. Sprinkle each breadsticks evenly with the parmesan cheese and salt.
5. Bake for 20 minutes or until turns crisp to your satisfaction.
6. Take it out and allow to cool down on a wired rack for at least 10-20 minutes. Serve and enjoy.

NUTRITIONAL VALUES (PER SERVING):

Calories:174
F:13g C:5g Fi:2g P:7g

Cheese Burst Breadsticks

Servings:
10

Preparation Time:
35-40 mins

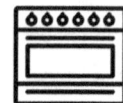

Method:
Bake

INGREDIENTS:

4 eggs, beaten

¼ cup butter, melted

2 Tablespoons cream cheese

1 ⅓ cup almond flour

½ teaspoon baking powder

3 cups shredded mozzarella cheese

¾ cup grated parmesan cheese

1 ½ teaspoon Italian herb blend (dried)

DIRECTIONS:

1. Preheat an oven to 400ºF-204ºC. Prepare a baking sheet by lining it with a parchment paper. Grease it with some coconut oil or butter. (You can also use coconut oil cooking spray to grease)
2. In a mixing bowl, whisk the eggs, butter, and cream cheese; combine well.
3. In another bowl, combine the almond flour, baking powder, and 1 teaspoon Italian herbs. Add 2 cups mozzarella cheese and 1/2 cup parmesan cheese; continue to mix.
4. Combine both mixtures with each other. Combine well until a well-combined dough is formed without any visible lumps.
5. Place the prepared breadstick dough over a lined baking sheet. Using your hands, press it to shape into a rectangle. Sprinkle evenly with remaining parmesan cheese, mozzarella cheese, and Italian herb blend.
6. Bake for 8 minutes.
7. Take a pizza cutter and make cuts to make breadsticks of your size. Bake for 7-8 more minutes or until turns crisp to your satisfaction.
8. Take it out and allow to cool down on a wired rack for at least 10-20 minutes. Serve and enjoy.

NUTRITIONAL VALUES (PER SERVING):

Calories: 212
F:18g C:4g fi:0.5g P:15g

Sesame Seed Breadsticks

Servings:
4-5

Preparation Time:
30-40 mins

Method:
Bake

INGREDIENTS:

1 Tablespoon olive oil (extra virgin)

1 medium egg white

¼ cup almond or coconut flour

1 teaspoon Himalayan pink salt

½ teaspoon sesame seeds

DIRECTIONS:

1. Preheat an oven to 325°F-162°C. Prepare a baking sheet by lining it with a parchment paper. Grease it with some coconut oil or butter. (You can also use coconut oil cooking spray to grease)
2. Beat the egg white in a mixing bowl.
3. Add the ½ teaspoon salt, ½ Tablespoon olive oil, and flour in another mixing bowl.
4. Combine both mixtures with each other. Combine well until a well-combined dough is formed without any visible lumps.
5. Place the prepared breadstick dough over a lined baking sheet. Using your hands, press it to shape into a rectangle. Coat it with remaining olive oil, salt and sesame seeds.
6. Take a pizza cutter and make cuts to prepare unbaked breadsticks.
7. Bake for 20 minutes or until turns crisp to your satisfaction.
8. Take it out and allow to cool down on a wired rack for at least 10-20 minutes. Serve and enjoy.

NUTRITIONAL VALUES (PER SERVING):

Calories:236
F:16g C:6g Fi:1g P:13g

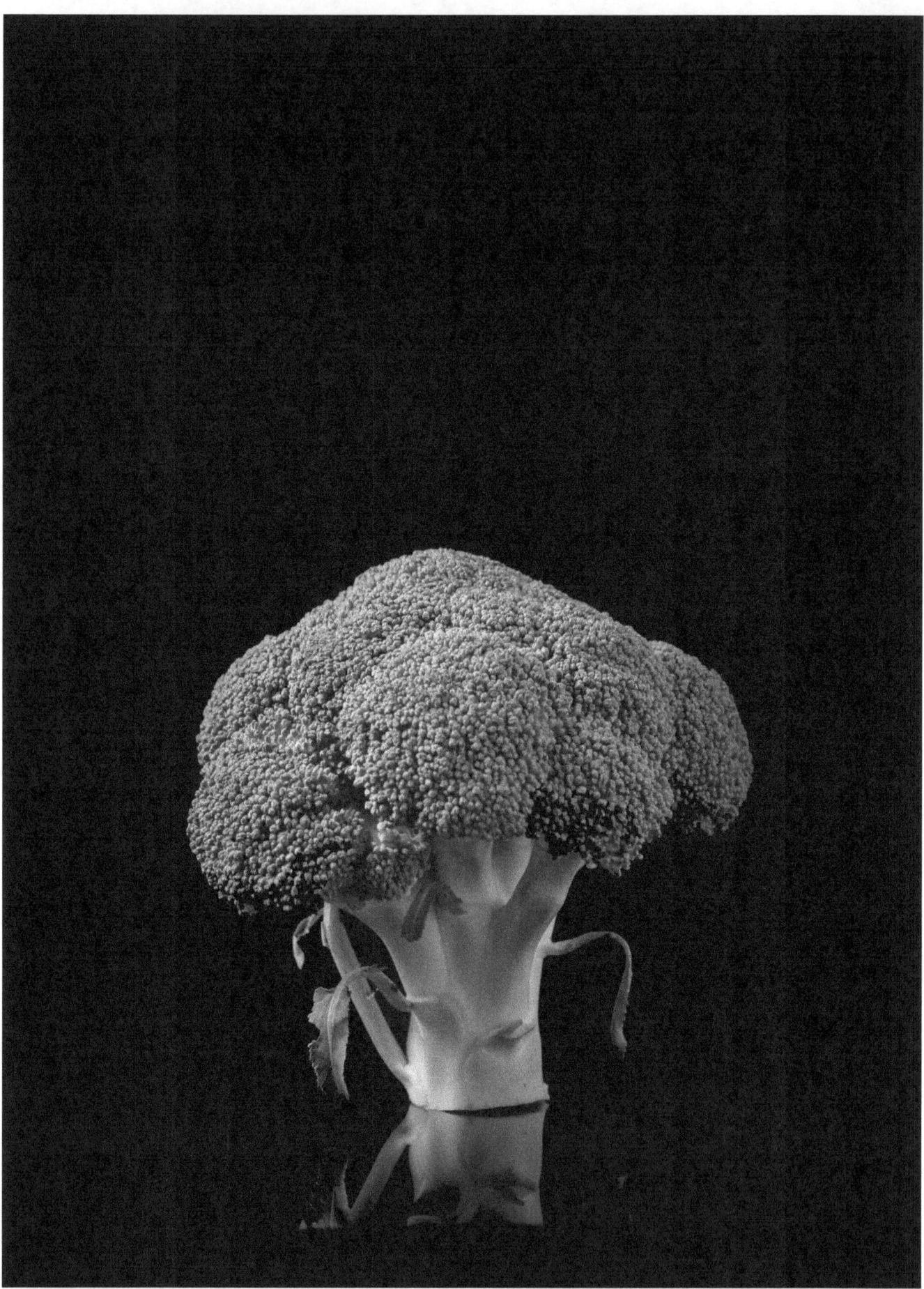

Broccoli Cheese Breadsticks

Servings:
8

Preparation Time:
30-40 mins

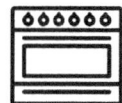

Method:
Bake

INGREDIENTS:

10 ounces broccoli florets

2 eggs, beaten

1 teaspoon onion powder

1 teaspoon garlic powder

1 teaspoon Italian herb blend (dried)

1 ¼ cup shredded mild cheddar cheese

½ cup grated parmesan cheese

1 Tablespoon butter, melted

DIRECTIONS:

1. Preheat an oven to 375°F-190°C. Prepare a baking sheet by lining it with a parchment paper. Grease it with some coconut oil or butter. (You can also use coconut oil cooking spray to grease)
2. In a blender, blend the broccoli florets until turn crumbly.
3. Beat the egg in a mixing bowl.
4. Add the blended broccoli, beaten eggs, 1 cup cheddar cheese, parmesan cheese, onion powder, garlic powder, and Italian herb in a mixing bowl.
5. Place the prepared breadstick mixture over a lined baking sheet. Using your hands, press it to shape into a rectangle.
6. Bake for 15 minutes. Take a pizza cutter and make cuts to prepare unbaked breadsticks.
7. Brush them with the butter. Sprinkle each breadsticks evenly with remaining cheddar cheese.
8. Bake for 5 more minutes or until turns crisp to your satisfaction.
9. Take it out and allow to cool down on a wired rack for at least 10-20 minutes. Serve and enjoy.

NUTRITIONAL VALUES (PER SERVING):

Calories:102
F:7g C:1g Fi:0g P:6g

Cheesy Cheddar Breadsticks

Servings:
8-10

Preparation Time:
30-40 mins

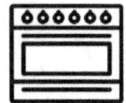

Method:
Bake

INGREDIENTS:

¾ cup almond flour

3 Tablespoons cream cheese

1 large egg

2 cups mozzarella cheese, shredded

1 Tablespoon psyllium husk powder

1 teaspoon baking powder

Flavorings:

3 ounces cheddar cheese

¼ cup parmesan cheese

1 teaspoon garlic powder

1 teaspoon onion powder

DIRECTIONS:

1. Preheat an oven to 400°F-204°C. Prepare a baking sheet by lining it with a parchment paper. Grease it with some coconut oil or butter. (You can also use coconut oil cooking spray to grease)
2. Beat the egg and cream cheese in a mixing bowl. Combine the almond flour, psyllium husk powder and baking powder in another mixing bowl.
3. In a heatproof bowl, add the mozzarella cheese. Microwave until melts completely. Add it with the egg mix and combine well.
4. Combine both mixtures with each other. Combine well until a well-combined dough is formed without any visible lumps.
5. Place the prepared breadstick dough over a lined baking sheet. Using your hands, press it to shape into a rectangle. Take a pizza cutter and make cuts to prepare unbaked breadsticks.
6. Top each breadsticks evenly with the flavorings.
7. Bake for 15 minutes or until turns crisp to your satisfaction.
8. Take it out and allow to cool down on a wired rack for at least 10-20 minutes. Serve and enjoy.

NUTRITIONAL VALUES (PER SERVING):

Calories: 257
F: 21g C: 6g Fi: 3g P: 17g

Cauliflower Spice Breadsticks

Servings:
8-10

Preparation Time:
30-40 mins

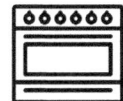

Method:
Bake

INGREDIENTS:

1 ½ cups Monterey jack cheese (grated)

½ teaspoon sage (ground)

½ teaspoon oregano (ground)

½ teaspoon thyme (dried)

¼ teaspoon mustard (ground)

2 large eggs (beaten)

1 ½ cups cauliflower rice

Ground black pepper to taste

DIRECTIONS:

1. Combine the cauliflower rice with some olive oil in a heatproof bowl; cook for 10 minutes in a microwave. Drain over paper and set aside.
2. Preheat an oven to 425°F-232°C. Prepare a baking sheet by lining it with a parchment paper. Grease it with some coconut oil or butter. (You can also use coconut oil cooking spray to grease)
3. Add the oregano, sage, thyme, cauliflower rice, 3 Tablespoon cheese, and mustard in a mixing bowl. Combine well.
4. Beat the egg with black pepper in another mixing bowl.
5. Combine both mixtures with each other. Combine well until a well-combined dough is formed without any visible lumps.
6. Place the prepared breadstick dough over a lined baking sheet. Using your hands, press it to shape into a rectangle. Take a pizza cutter and make cuts to prepare unbaked breadsticks.
7. Bake for 10 minutes. Sprinkle each breadsticks evenly with remaining cheese.
8. Bake for 5 more minutes or until turns crisp to your satisfaction.
9. Take it out and allow to cool down on a wired rack for at least 10-20 minutes. Serve and enjoy.

NUTRITIONAL VALUES (PER SERVING):

Calories:113
F:9g C:2g Fi:0g P:7g

CHAPTER 7
KETO CAKES

Cinnamon Bundt Cake

Servings:
4-5

Preparation Time:
50-55 mins

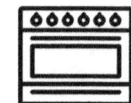

Method:
Bake

INGREDIENTS:

1 ½ cups almond flour

5 large eggs

½ teaspoon Stevia granular (adjust more or less to taste)

1 pinch salt

½ cup melted butter

1 teaspoon cinnamon

½ cup powdered erythritol

½ cup unsweetened almond milk

DIRECTIONS:

1. Preheat an oven to 350ºF-176ºC. Prepare a medium-size Bundt cake pan by greasing it with some coconut oil or butter. (You can also use coconut oil cooking spray to grease)
2. In a mixing bowl, beat the eggs, butter, and almond milk.
3. In another bowl, combine the almond flour, and erythritol, stevia, salt, and cinnamon. Stir until smooth.
4. Combine both mixtures with each other. Combine well until smooth batter is formed without any visible lumps.
5. Take the prepared cake batter and slowly pour it in the greased pan. Smoothen the top using a spatula or spoon.
6. Place the pan in the preheated oven and bake for 30-35 minutes or until turns golden brown. You can check by inserting a toothpick; when the bread is baked well, toothpick comes out clean.
7. Take out the pan and allow it to cool down on a wired rack for at least 30 minutes. Shake the pan gently and take out the prepared cake.
8. Cut into slices and serve!

NUTRITIONAL VALUES (PER SERVING):

Calories:136
F:12g C:2g Fi:0g P:8g

Keto Milk Cake

Servings:
6-8

Preparation Time:
20 mins

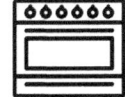
Method:
Bake

INGREDIENTS:

14 eggs, separated

1 cube butter, melted

1 ½ cup almond or coconut milk

1 ¾ cup coconut flour

1 ½ teaspoons baking soda

2 teaspoons vanilla extract

2-3 teaspoon liquid Stevia (adjust less or more to taste)

DIRECTIONS:

1. Preheat an oven to 350°F-176°C. Prepare a medium-size cake pan by greasing it with some coconut oil or butter. (You can also use coconut oil cooking spray to grease)
2. Beat the whites until turns stiff in a mixing bowl. In another bowl, whisk the yolks and stevia until frothy. Mix in the milk, melted butter, and vanilla. Add the egg whites and whisk well.
3. In another bowl, combine all dry ingredients.
4. Combine both mixtures with each other. Combine well until smooth batter is formed without any visible lumps.
5. Take the prepared cake batter and slowly pour it in the greased pan. Smoothen the top using a spatula or spoon.
6. Place the pan in the preheated oven and bake for 25 minutes or until turns golden brown. You can check by inserting a toothpick; when the bread is baked well, toothpick comes out clean.
7. Take out the pan and allow it to cool down on a wired rack for at least 30 minutes. Shake the pan gently and take out the prepared cake.
8. Cut into slices and serve!

NUTRITIONAL VALUES (PER SERVING):

Calories:168
F:12g C:5g Fi:0g P:6g

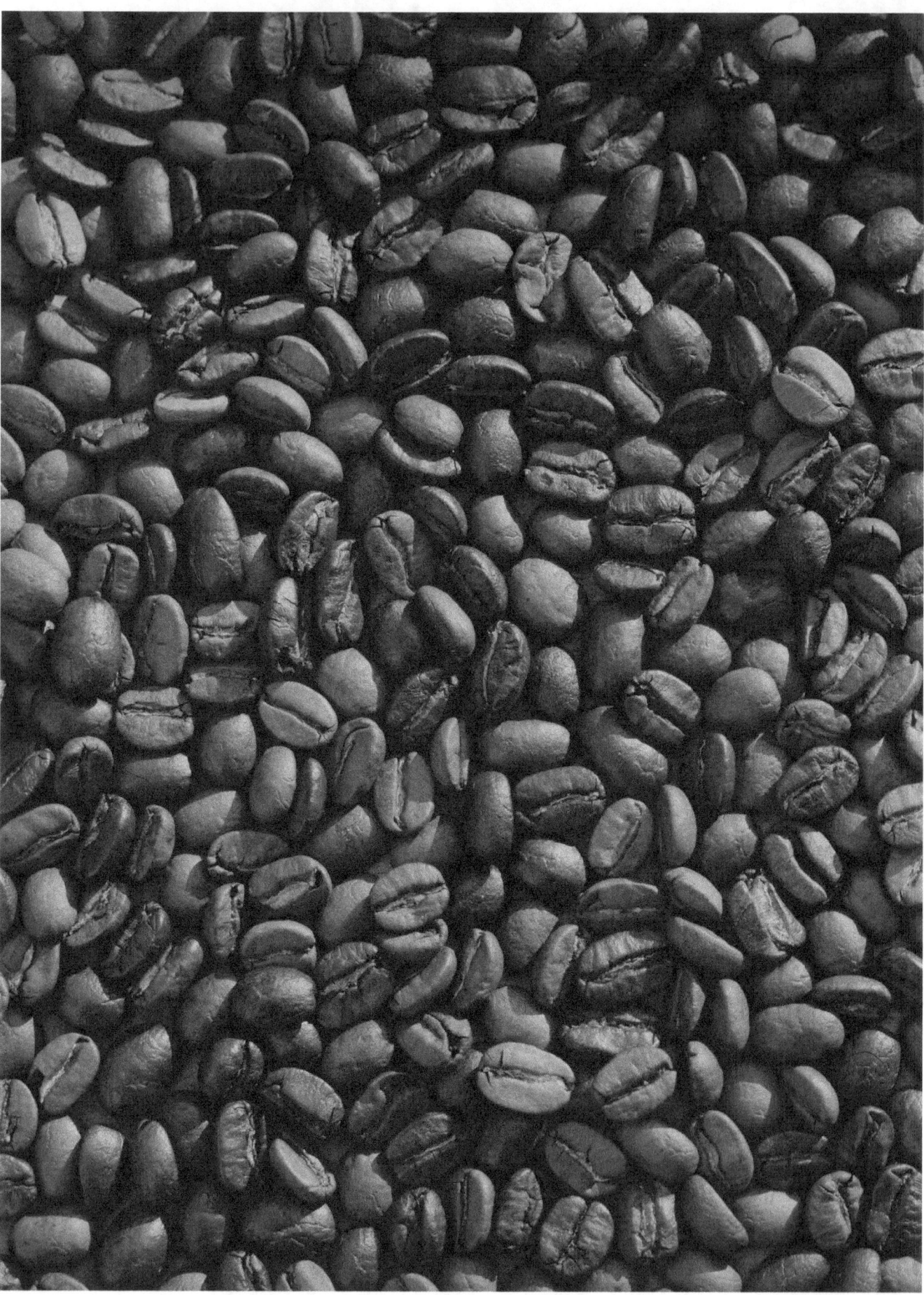

Spiced Brownie Cake

Servings:
2

Preparation Time:
5-10 mins

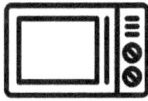

Method:
Microwave

INGREDIENTS:

¼ cup cacao powder

¼ cup brewed coffee, unsweetened and cooled

¼ cup coconut oil

1 teaspoon baking powder

2 large squares unsweetened dark chocolate (grated)

1 large egg

4 Tablespoons Erythritol

2 Tablespoons chia seeds (ground)

½ teaspoon cinnamon

Pinch of sea salt

DIRECTIONS:

1. Grease two mugs with some coconut oil or butter. (You can also use coconut oil cooking spray to grease)
2. Add the grated chocolate and dry ingredients in a mixing bowl. Combine well.
3. Beat the egg, coconut oil and coffee in another mixing bowl. Mix well.
4. Combine both mixtures with each other. Combine well until smooth batter is formed without any visible lumps.
5. Add the mixture between 2 mugs.
6. Microwave on high temperature setting for 90 seconds.
7. Cool down for a while and serve!

NUTRITIONAL VALUES (PER SERVING):

Calories: 308
F: 31g C: 12g fi: 6g P: 9g

Cacao Zucchini Cakes

Servings:
70-80

Preparation Time:
14-16 mins

Method:
Bake

INGREDIENTS:

6 large eggs

2 ¾ cups almond flour

2 teaspoons baking powder

2 teaspoons vanilla extract, unsweetened

1 1/3 cups Erythritol (powdered)

½ cup butter (melted)

½ cup cacao powder

½ teaspoon sea salt

2 medium zucchini, peeled and cubed

Frosting:

¼ cup coconut oil

½ cup cacao powder

Stevia drops to taste

DIRECTIONS:

1. Puree the zucchini in a blender. Set aside.
2. Preheat an oven to 325°F-162°C. Prepare a Bundt pan by greasing it with some coconut oil or butter. (You can also use coconut oil cooking spray to grease)
3. Mix the dry ingredients in a mixing bowl. Beat the eggs, butter, vanilla extract and puree in another mixing bowl.
4. Combine both mixtures with each other. Combine well until smooth batter is formed without any visible lumps.
5. Take the prepared cake batter and slowly pour it in the greased pan. Smoothen the top using a spatula or spoon.
6. Place the pan in the preheated oven and bake for 50 minutes or until turns golden brown. You can check by inserting a toothpick; when the bread is baked well, toothpick comes out clean.
7. Take out the pan and allow it to cool down on a wired rack for at least 30 minutes. Shake the pan gently and take out the prepared cake.
8. Combine the cacao powder and coconut oil in a heat safe bowl. Melt in a microwave until combine well. Mix in the stevia to taste. Spread it over the cake.
9. Cut into slices and serve!

NUTRITIONAL VALUES (PER SERVING):

Calories:194
F:21g C:8g fi:3g P:7g

Dessert Choco Cake

Servings:
8-10

Preparation Time:
40-50 mins

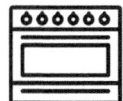

Method:
Bake

INGREDIENTS:

Dry ingredients:

2 cups ground flax seed

½ cup almonds, ground

½ cup pumpkin seeds, ground

4 teaspoons baking powder

½ teaspoon salt

½ cup cocoa powder

1 ½ to 2 teaspoon liquid Stevia

Wet ingredients:

6 eggs, beaten

½ cup sour cream

1 tablespoon vanilla extract

1 cup canola oil

1 cup half & half cream

DIRECTIONS:

1. Preheat an oven to 350°F-176°C. Prepare a medium-size cake pan by greasing it with some coconut oil or butter. (You can also use coconut oil cooking spray to grease)
2. Combine dry ingredients in a mixing bowl.
3. Beat the eggs and other wet ingredients in another bowl.
4. Combine both mixtures with each other. Combine well until smooth batter is formed without any visible lumps.
5. Take the prepared cake batter and slowly pour it in the greased pan. Smoothen the top using a spatula or spoon.
6. Place the pan in the preheated oven and bake for 30 minutes or until turns golden brown. You can check by inserting a toothpick: when the bread is baked well, toothpick comes out clean.
7. Take out the pan and allow it to cool down on a wired rack for at least 30 minutes. Shake the pan gently and take out the prepared cake.
8. Cut into slices and serve!

NUTRITIONAL VALUES (PER SERVING):

Calories:107
F:12g C:3g fi:0g P:4g

Keto Sweet Cheese

		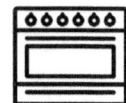
Servings: 6	Preparation Time: 60 mins	Method: Bake

INGREDIENTS:

4 ounce cream cheese, softened

1/2 cup butter softened

1 ½ to 2 teaspoon liquid Stevia

5 eggs, beaten

1 teaspoon vanilla extract

1 teaspoon lemon extract

1 ½ cups + 2 Tablespoons almond flour

1 teaspoon baking powder

A dash of salt

DIRECTIONS:

1. Preheat an oven to 350°F-176°C. Prepare a medium-size Bundt pan by greasing it with some coconut oil or butter. (You can also use coconut oil cooking spray to grease)
2. Whisk the butter, cream cheese and Stevia in a mixing bowl. Add the beaten eggs, both extracts and combine well.
3. Mix the almond flour, salt, and baking powder in another mixing bowl.
4. Combine both mixtures with each other. Combine well until smooth batter is formed without any visible lumps.
5. Take the prepared cake batter and slowly pour it in the greased pan. Smoothen the top using a spatula or spoon.
6. Place the pan in the preheated oven and bake for 50-55 minutes or until turns golden brown. You can check by inserting a toothpick; when the bread is baked well, toothpick comes out clean.
7. Take out the pan and allow it to cool down on a wired rack for at least 30 minutes. Shake the pan gently and take out the prepared cake.
8. Cut into slices and serve!

NUTRITIONAL VALUES (PER SERVING):

Calories:286
F:28g C:4g Fi:0g P:11g

Pumpkin Almond Cake

Servings:
12-14

Preparation Time:
20 mins

Method:
Bake

INGREDIENTS:

6 large eggs

½ cup butter, melted

2 teaspoons baking powder

2 teaspoons pumpkin pie spice

2 ¾ cups almond flour

1 1/3 cups Erythritol (powdered)

2 teaspoons vanilla extract, unsweetened

½ teaspoon sea salt

8 ½ ounces pumpkin (puree)

Glaze:

1 teaspoon vanilla extract, unsweetened

½ cup Erythritol (powdered)

¼ cup butter

1 teaspoon cinnamon

NUTRITIONAL VALUES (PER SERVING):

Calories:204
F:25g C:8g Fi:2g P:9g

DIRECTIONS:

1. Preheat an oven to 325°F-162°C. Prepare a medium-size cake pan by greasing it with some coconut oil or butter. (You can also use coconut oil cooking spray to grease)
2. Combine the dry ingredients a mixing bowl. Beat the eggs, butter, vanilla extract and pumpkin puree in another mixing bowl.
3. Combine both mixtures with each other. Combine well until smooth batter is formed without any visible lumps.
4. Take the prepared cake batter and slowly pour it in the greased pan. Smoothen the top using a spatula or spoon.
5. Place the pan in the preheated oven and bake for 55-60 minutes or until turns golden brown. You can check by inserting a toothpick; when the bread is baked well, toothpick comes out clean.
6. Take out the pan and allow it to cool down on a wired rack for at least 30 minutes. Shake the pan gently and take out the prepared cake.
7. Combine the butter, cinnamon and vanilla extract in a heat safe bowl. Melt in a microwave until combine well. Mix in the stevia to taste. Spread it over the cake. Sprinkle with some powdered Erythritol on top.
8. Cut into slices and serve!

Coconut Spiced Mug Cakes

Servings:
1

Preparation Time:
5-10 mins

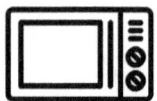

Method:
Microwave

INGREDIENTS:

- 1 large egg
- 2 Tablespoons Erythritol
- 1 Tablespoon coconut oil
- 2 Tablespoons almond flour
- 1 Tablespoon coconut flour
- ½ teaspoon rum extract
- ⅛ teaspoon baking soda
- ⅛ teaspoon nutmeg (ground)
- ¼ teaspoon cinnamon (ground)

DIRECTIONS:

1. Grease a mug with some coconut oil or butter. (You can also use coconut oil cooking spray to grease)
2. In a mixing bowl, combine the almond flour, coconut flour, Erythritol, cinnamon, baking soda and nutmeg. Combine well.
3. In another bowl, beat the egg, coconut oil and rum extract. Mix well.
4. Combine both mixtures with each other. Combine well until smooth batter is formed without any visible lumps.
5. Add the mixture in the mug.
6. Microwave on high temperature setting for 90 seconds.
7. Cool down for a while and serve!

NUTRITIONAL VALUES (PER SERVING):

Calories: 297
F:29g C:8g fi:2g P:6g

Keto Spice Mug Cake

  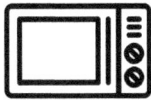

Servings: 1

Preparation Time: 15-20 mins

Method: Microwave

INGREDIENTS:

1 Tablespoon Erythritol

1 Tablespoon extra-virgin olive oil or coconut oil

1 large egg

2 Tablespoons almond flour

1 Tablespoon coconut flour

½ teaspoon cinnamon (ground)

⅛ teaspoon baking soda

DIRECTIONS:

1. Grease a mug with some coconut oil or butter. (You can also use coconut oil cooking spray to grease)
2. In a mixing bowl, combine the dry ingredients. Combine well.
3. In another bowl, beat the egg, and coconut oil. Mix well.
4. Combine both mixtures with each other. Combine well until smooth batter is formed without any visible lumps.
5. Add the mixture in the mug.
6. Microwave on high temperature setting for 90 seconds.
7. Cool down for a while and serve!

NUTRITIONAL VALUES (PER SERVING):

Calories: 284
F: 26g C: 9g Fi: 2g P: 12g

CHAPTER 8
KETO CRACKERS

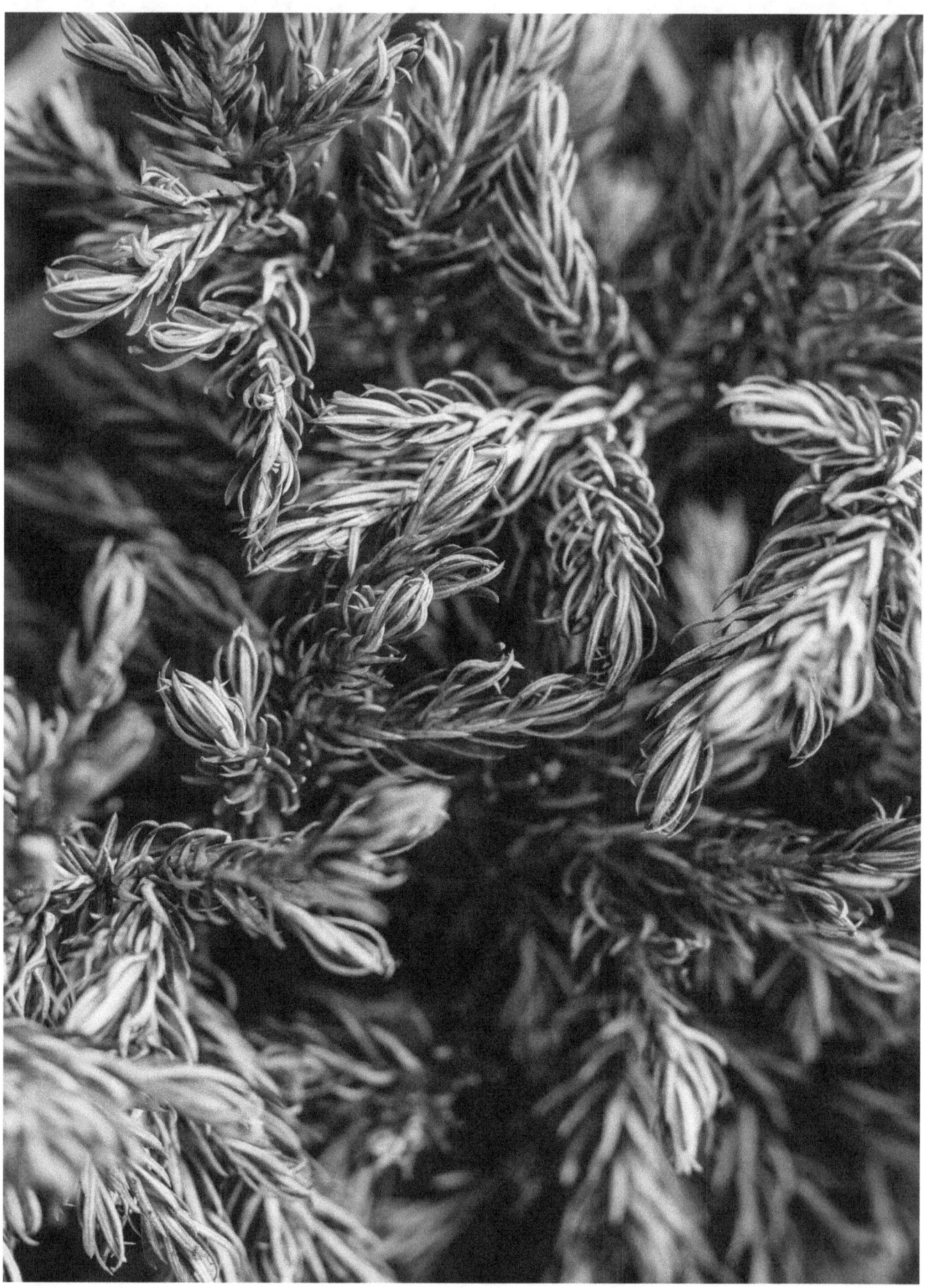

Goat Cheese Rosemary Crackers

Servings:
25-30

Preparation Time:
10 mins

Method:
Bake

INGREDIENTS:

4 Tablespoons butter, melted

6 ounces goat cheese

½ cup coconut flour

2 Tablespoons fresh rosemary, chopped

1 teaspoon baking powder

DIRECTIONS:

1. Preheat an oven to 375°F-190°C. Prepare two parchment papers by greasing with some coconut oil or butter. (You can also use coconut oil cooking spray to grease)
2. In a food processor or blender, combine all ingredients and process until smooth. Combine well until a round dough is formed.
3. Place the prepared cracker dough between two greased papers. Using a rolling pin, roll out the dough into an evenly thin layer (¼ or ½ inch thin).
4. Take a knife or cookie cutter, cut into crackers of your preferred size.
5. Place in the preheated oven and bake for 20 minutes or until turns crisp and light brown. Take out and allow it to cool down on a wired rack for at least 15-20 minutes.
6. Enjoy freshly baked crackers!

NUTRITIONAL VALUES (PER SERVING):

Calories: 103
F:8g C:2g Fi:0g P:4g

Spinach Chili Crackers

Servings:
16

Preparation Time:
50-60 mins

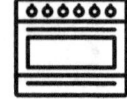

Method:
Bake

INGREDIENTS:

5 ounces spinach, chopped

1 ½ cups almond flour

¼ cup butter, melted

¼ cup coconut flour

½ cup flax meal

½ cup parmesan cheese (grated)

½ teaspoon chili peppers (dried and flaked)

½ teaspoon cumin (ground)

½ teaspoon salt

DIRECTIONS:

1. Preheat an oven to 400°F-204°C. Prepare two parchment papers by greasing with some coconut oil or butter. (You can also use coconut oil cooking spray to grease)
2. In a boiling water, wilt the spinach leaves until turn softened. Drain water, squeeze moisture from the leaves, and add the leaves in a mixing bowl. Add in a food processor, and blend until smooth.
3. In a mixing bowl, combine all the dry ingredients. Combine well. Mix in the spinach and butter.
4. Combine well until a round dough is formed. Cover with a plastic paper and refrigerate the mixture for 1 hour.
5. Place the prepared cracker dough between two greased papers. Using a rolling pin, roll out the dough into an evenly thin layer (¼ or ½ inch thin).
6. Take a knife or cookie cutter, cut into 16 crackers of your preferred size.
7. Place in the preheated oven and bake for 20 minutes or until turns crisp and light brown. Take out and allow it to cool down on a wired rack for at least 15-20 minutes.
8. Enjoy freshly baked crackers!

NUTRITIONAL VALUES (PER SERVING):

Calories:123
F:11g C:4g Fi:1g P:5g

Yummy Parmesan Crackers

Servings:
16

Preparation Time:
40-50 mins

Method:
Bake

INGREDIENTS:

1 cup water

½ cup flax meal

1 cup almond flour

1 cup parmesan cheese (grated)

2 Tablespoons whole psyllium husks

1 teaspoon salt

¼ teaspoon black pepper

DIRECTIONS:

1. Preheat an oven to 325°F-162°C. Prepare two parchment papers by greasing with some coconut oil or butter. (You can also use coconut oil cooking spray to grease)
2. In a mixing bowl, combine all the dry ingredients. Combine well and add the grated parmesan cheese; combine again.
3. Add water and mix well. Set aside for 15 minutes.
4. Combine well until a round dough is formed.
5. Place the prepared cracker dough between two greased papers. Using a rolling pin, roll out the dough into an evenly thin layer (¼ or ½ inch thin).
6. Take a knife or cookie cutter, cut into crackers of your preferred size.
7. Place in the preheated oven and bake for 40 minutes or until turns crisp and light brown. Take out and allow it to cool down on a wired rack for at least 15-20 minutes.
8. Enjoy freshly baked crackers!

NUTRITIONAL VALUES (PER SERVING):

Calories: 84
F:8g C:3g Fi:2g P:4g

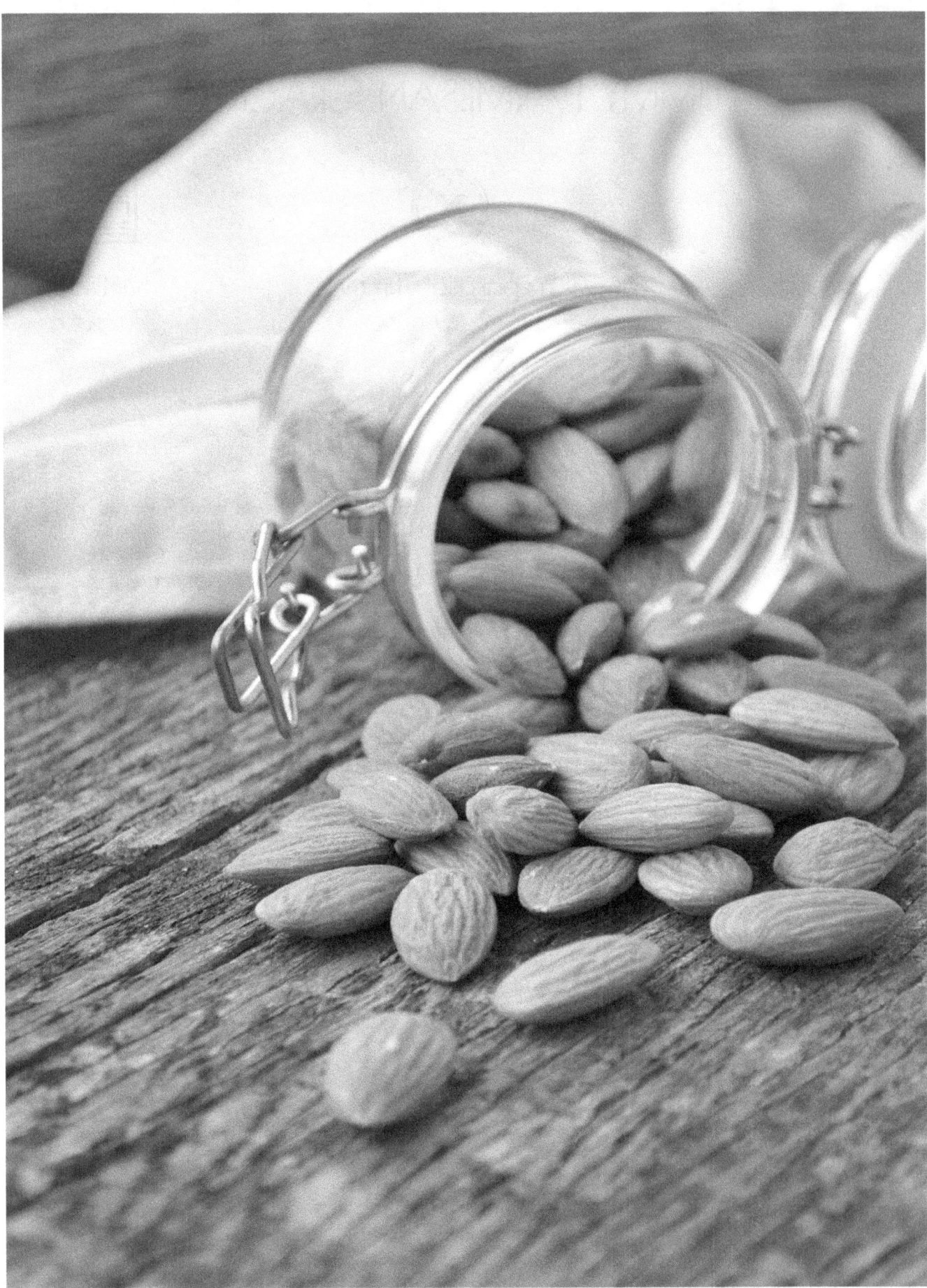

Rosemary Almond Crackers

Servings:
5-6

Preparation Time:
30-40 mins

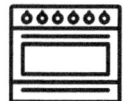
Method:
Bake

INGREDIENTS:

1 large egg

2 Tablespoons rosemary (chopped)

1 Tablespoon olive oil (extra virgin)

1 cup almonds (ground)

½ cup flax seeds (ground)

1 teaspoon baking soda

½ teaspoon onion powder

⅓ teaspoon black pepper

⅓ teaspoon sea salt

DIRECTIONS:

1. Preheat an oven to 350°F-176°C. Prepare two parchment papers by greasing with some coconut oil or butter. (You can also use coconut oil cooking spray to grease)
2. Beat the eggs and olive oil in a mixing bowl.
3. In a mixing bowl, combine all the dry ingredients. Combine well. Set aside for 15 minutes.
4. Combine both mixtures with each other. Combine well until a round dough is formed.
5. Place the prepared cracker dough between two greased papers. Using a rolling pin, roll out the dough into an evenly thin layer (¼ or ½ inch thin).
6. Take a knife or cookie cutter, cut into crackers of your preferred size.
7. Place in the preheated oven and bake for 15 minutes or until turns crisp and light brown. Take out and allow it to cool down on a wired rack for at least 15-20 minutes.
8. Enjoy freshly baked crackers!

NUTRITIONAL VALUES (PER SERVING):

Calories:112
F:9g C:5g fi:2g P:4g

Savory Seed Crackers

Servings:
40-45

Preparation Time:
70-80 mins

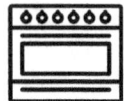

Method:
Bake

INGREDIENTS:

1 cup boiling water

1 Tablespoon psyllium powder

1 cup almond flour

1 teaspoon salt

¼ cup coconut oil

⅓ cup chia seeds

⅓ cup sunflower seeds

⅓ cup flax seed

⅓ cup pumpkin seeds

⅓ cup sesame seeds

DIRECTIONS:

1. Preheat an oven to 300°F-148°C. Prepare two parchment papers by greasing with some coconut oil or butter. (You can also use coconut oil cooking spray to grease)
2. Combine the coconut oil and water in a mixing bowl. Add remaining ingredients in a blender or food processor; pulse until ground.
3. Combine both mixtures with each other. Combine well until a round dough is formed.
4. Place the prepared cracker dough between two greased papers. Using a rolling pin, roll out the dough into an evenly thin layer (¼ or ½ inch thin).
5. Take a knife or cookie cutter, cut into crackers of your preferred size.
6. Place in the preheated oven and bake for 60 minutes or until turns crisp and light brown. Take out and allow it to cool down on a wired rack for at least 15-20 minutes.
7. Enjoy freshly baked crackers!

NUTRITIONAL VALUES (PER SERVING):

Calories:63
F:8g C:3g fi:0.5g P:2g

CHAPTER 9
KETO COOKIES

Cocolicious Cookies

Servings:
10-12

Preparation Time:
15-20 mins

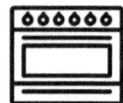
Method:
Bake

INGREDIENTS:

½ stick (2 ounce) butter, melted

2 Tablespoons coconut flour

2 egg whites

1 ½ cups coconut flakes

1 cup erythritol

DIRECTIONS:

1. Preheat an oven to 400°F-204°C. Prepare a baking sheet by lining it with a parchment paper. Grease it with some coconut oil or butter. (You can also use coconut oil cooking spray to grease)
2. Combine the flour, coconut flakes and erythritol in a mixing bowl.
3. Beat the egg whites and melted butter in another bowl.
4. Combine both mixtures with each other. Combine well until smooth batter is formed without any visible lumps.
5. Take the prepared batter and drop a spoonful over the greased sheet. Keep some space between each drop.
6. Place in the preheated oven and bake for 50 minutes or until turns golden brown. Take out the sheet and allow it to cool down on a wired rack for at least 30 minutes.
7. Enjoy warm cookies!

NUTRITIONAL VALUES (PER SERVING):

Calories:136
F:12g C:2g fi:0g P:4g

Pumpkin Cookies

Servings:
12-14

Preparation Time:
50-60 mins

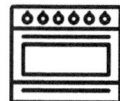

Method:
Bake

INGREDIENTS:

1 cup almond flour

1 cup almonds, ground

1 egg white

1 cup pumpkin purée

10-15 drops liquid Stevia

¼ cup coconut flakes

¼ cup lemon zest, grated

DIRECTIONS:

1. Preheat an oven to 300°F-148°C. Prepare a baking sheet by lining it with a parchment paper. Grease it with some coconut oil or butter. (You can also use coconut oil cooking spray to grease)
2. Combine the flour, almonds, coconut flakes and lemon zest in a mixing bowl.
3. In another bowl, whisk the egg white until foamy. Add remaining ingredient and combine well.
4. Combine both mixtures with each other. Combine well until smooth batter is formed without any visible lumps.
5. Take the prepared batter and drop a spoonful over the greased sheet. Keep some space between each drop.
6. Place in the preheated oven and bake for 25-30 minutes or until turns golden brown. Take out the sheet and allow it to cool down on a wired rack for at least 30 minutes.
7. Enjoy warm cookies!

NUTRITIONAL VALUES (PER SERVING):

Calories:292
F:20g C:9g Fi:3g P:8g

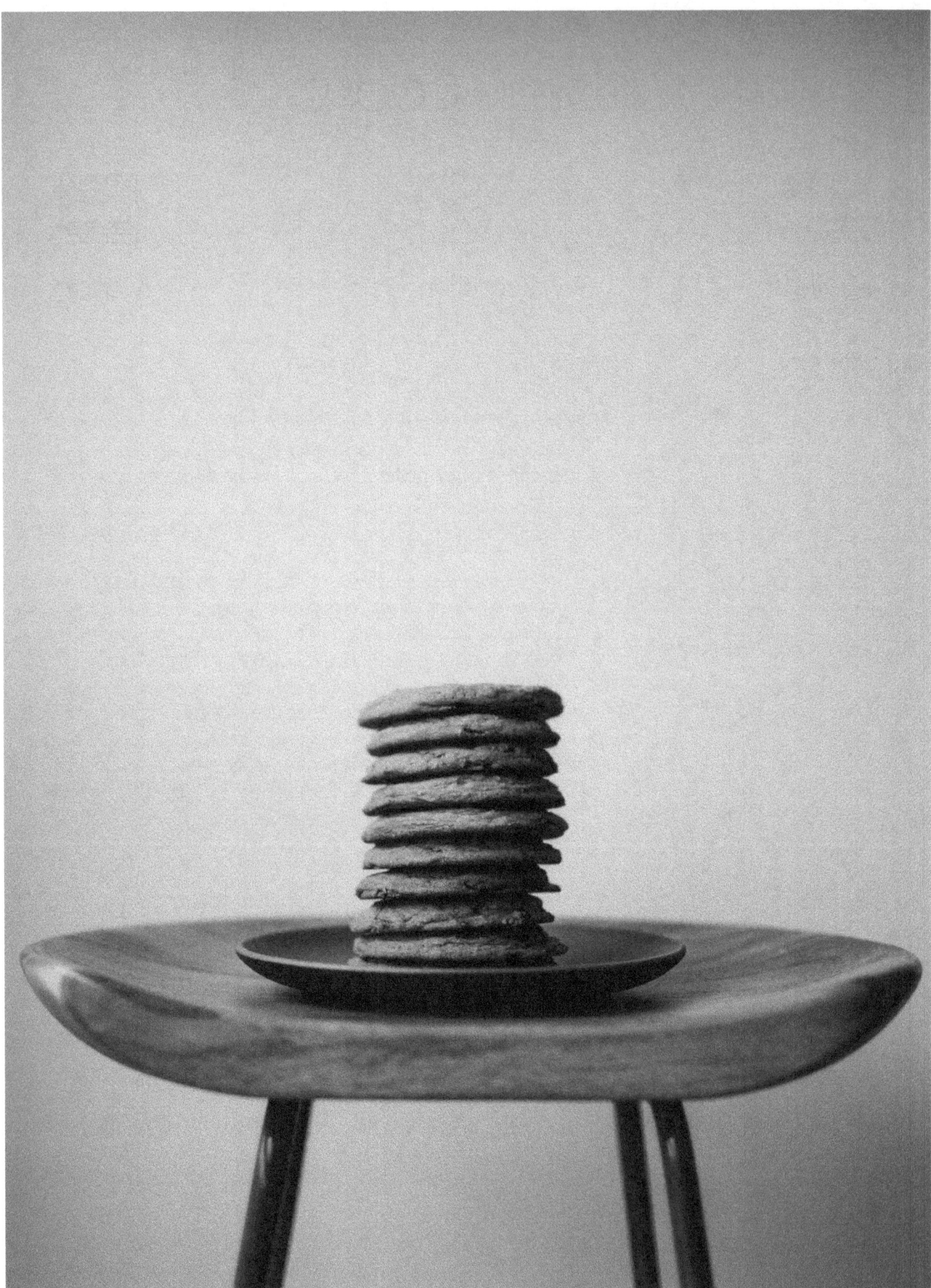

Chocolate Chip Cookies

Servings:
12

Preparation Time:
25-30 mins

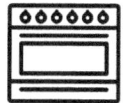
Method:
Bake

INGREDIENTS:

¾ cup Erythritol

1 ½ cups almond flour

½ cup salted butter, melted

1 teaspoon vanilla extract

1 egg, beaten

½ teaspoon baking powder

¼ teaspoon salt

½ teaspoon xanthan gum (optional)

¾ cup unsweetened chocolate chips

DIRECTIONS:

1. Preheat an oven to 350°F-176°C. Prepare a baking sheet by lining it with a parchment paper. Grease it with some coconut oil or butter. (You can also use coconut oil cooking spray to grease)
2. Beat the eggs in a mixing bowl; add the butter, Erythritol, vanilla extract and combine well.
3. Combine the almond flour, xanthan gum, baking powder and salt in another bowl.
4. Combine both mixtures with each other. Combine well until smooth batter is formed without any visible lumps. Mix in the chocolate chips.
5. Take the prepared batter and drop a spoonful over the greased sheet. Keep some space between each drop.
6. Place in the preheated oven and bake for 10-12 minutes or until turns golden brown. Take out the sheet and allow it to cool down on a wired rack for at least 30 minutes.
7. Enjoy warm cookies!

NUTRITIONAL VALUES (PER SERVING):

Calories:168
F:16g C:2g Fi:0g P:5g

Almond Cream Cookies

Servings:
20-24

Preparation Time:
25-30 mins

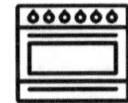

Method:
Bake

INGREDIENTS:

3 cups almond flour

2 ounces cream cheese

1 egg white

¼ cup butter, melted

2 teaspoon vanilla extract

¾ cup erythritol

DIRECTIONS:

1. Preheat an oven to 350ºF-176ºC. Prepare a baking sheet by lining it with a parchment paper. Grease it with some coconut oil or butter. (You can also use coconut oil cooking spray to grease)
2. Beat the egg white in a mixing bowl, add the butter, cream cheese, and erythritol and combine well.
3. Combine the flour and vanilla extract in another bowl.
4. Combine both mixtures with each other. Combine well until smooth batter is formed without any visible lumps.
5. Take the prepared batter and drop a spoonful over the greased sheet. Keep some space between each drop.
6. Place in the preheated oven and bake for 15 minutes or until turns golden brown. Take out the sheet and allow it to cool down on a wired rack for at least 30 minutes.
7. Enjoy warm cookies!

NUTRITIONAL VALUES (PER SERVING):

Calories:111
F:7g C:3g fi:0g P:3g

CONCLUSION

The revolutionary ketogenic diet has been around for many decades and is aimed at promoting healthy weight loss and improved holistic health by minimizing the consumption of bad carbohydrates and increasing the consumption of healthy fats instead.

I truly believe that the need to adapt to a smart diet, is greater now than ever. I myself have experienced health hazarding effects relying on a high carbohydrate diet and found switching to Keto a wonderful experience.

Breads form a very crucial part of our everyday diet. I have encountered many people choosing not to switch to the keto diet thinking that they have to give up on everyday breads. Contrary to such belief, keto breads can be prepared in many different varieties fulfilling any of those carb cravings.

I sincerely hope you enjoyed this book and found it encouraging to learn how to prepare various keto breads, and discover it is not as daunting a task as it seems.

Lastly, if you enjoyed this book, please take the time to review it on Amazon. Your honest feedback would be greatly appreciated.

Best of luck on your Keto journey!